Antidepressants - Preclinical, Clinical and Translational Aspects

Edited by Berend Olivier

Published in London, United Kingdom

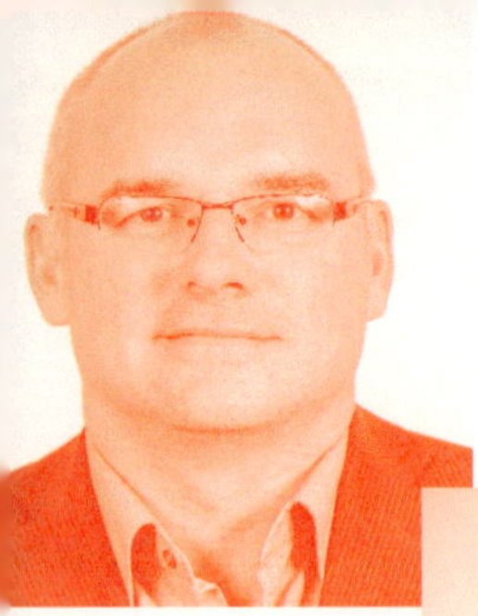
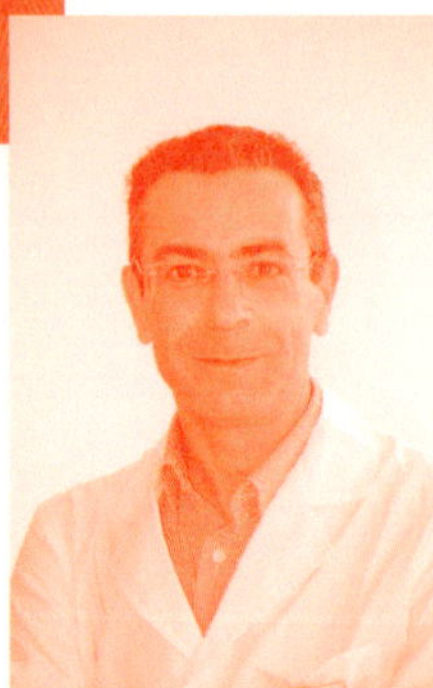
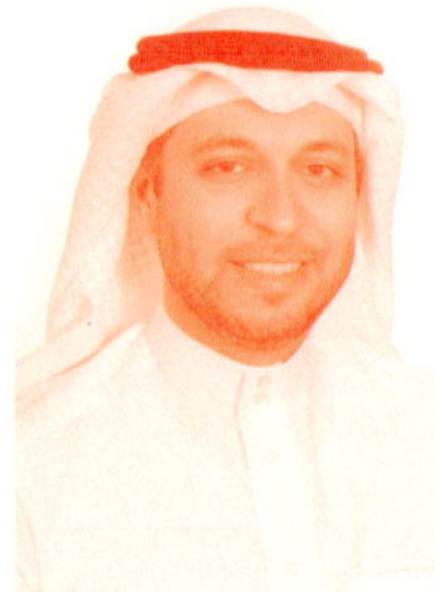
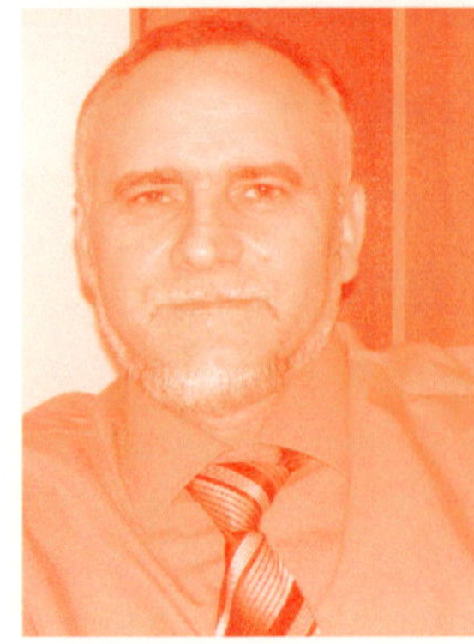
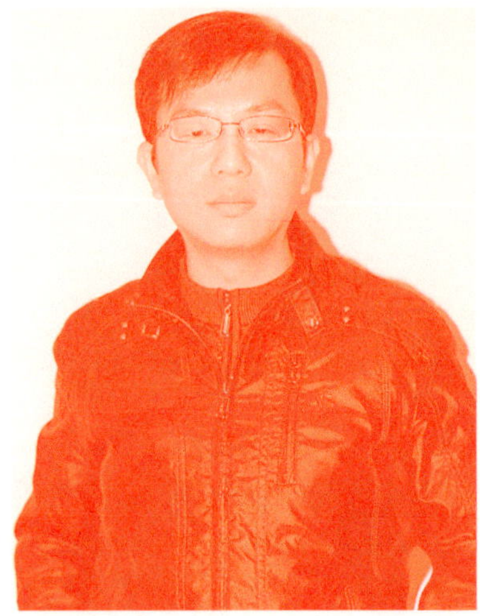
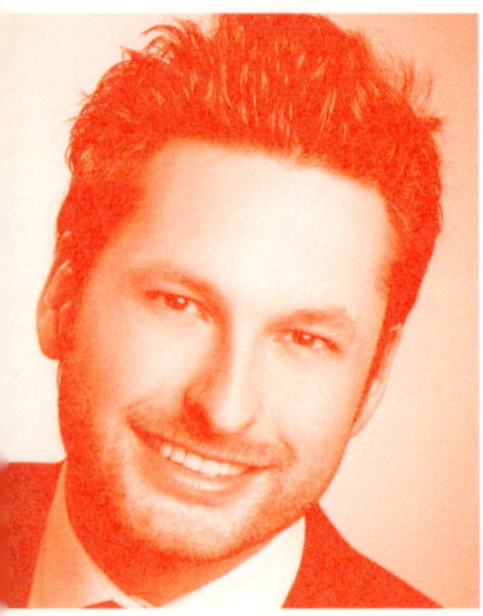
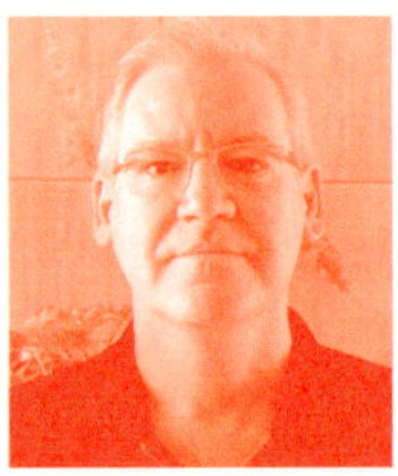

IntechOpen

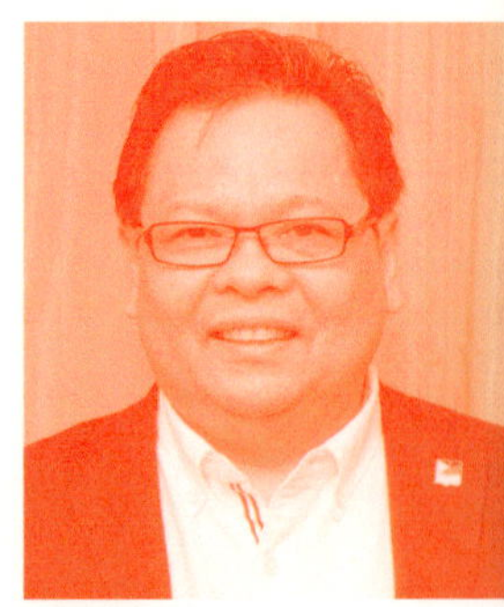
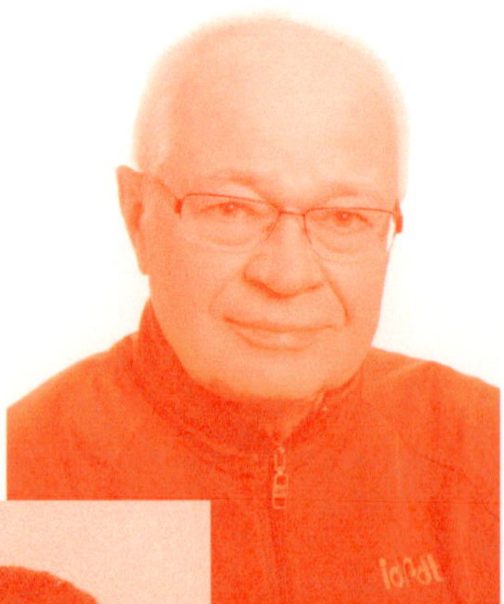
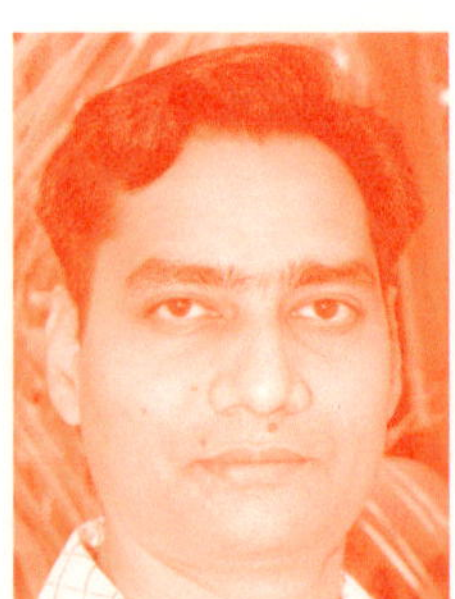
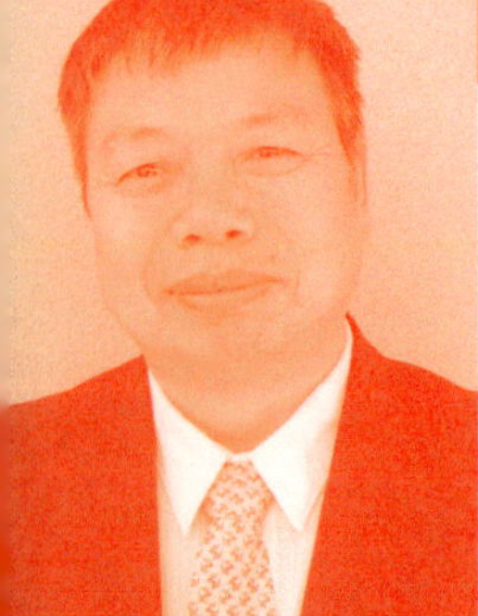
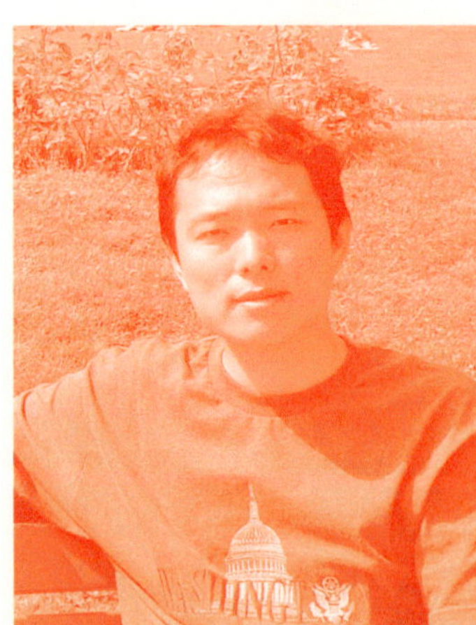
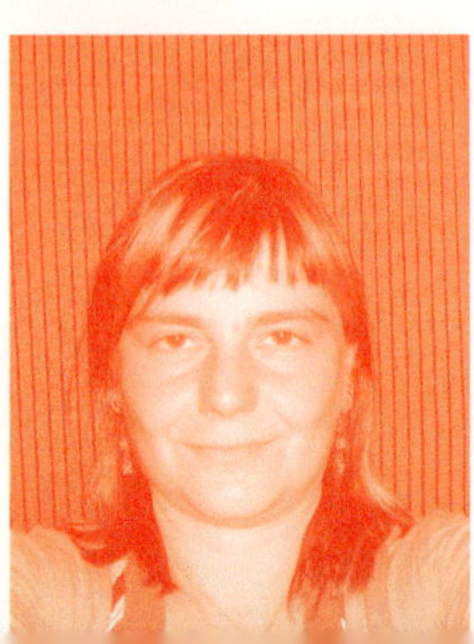

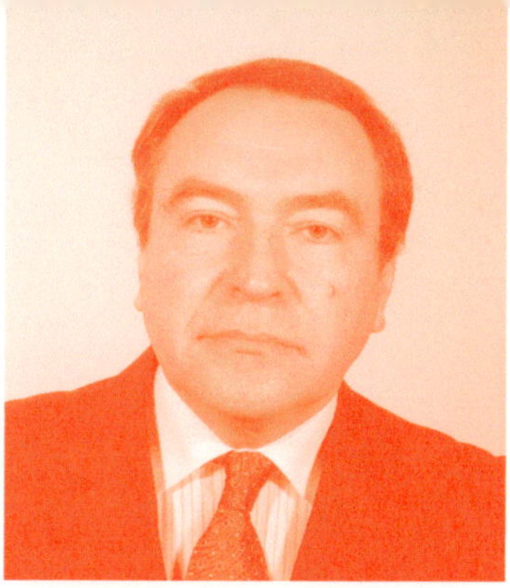
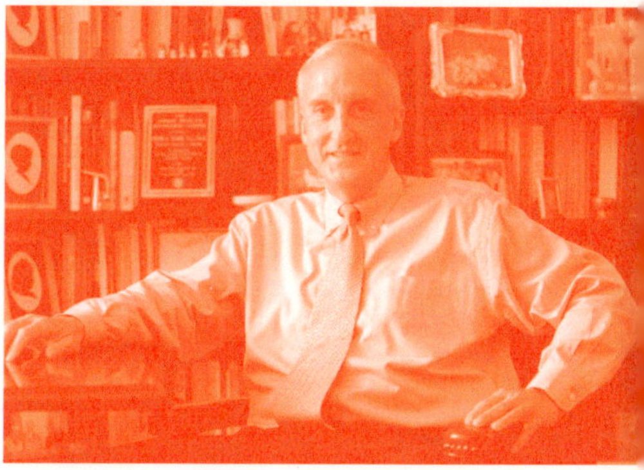
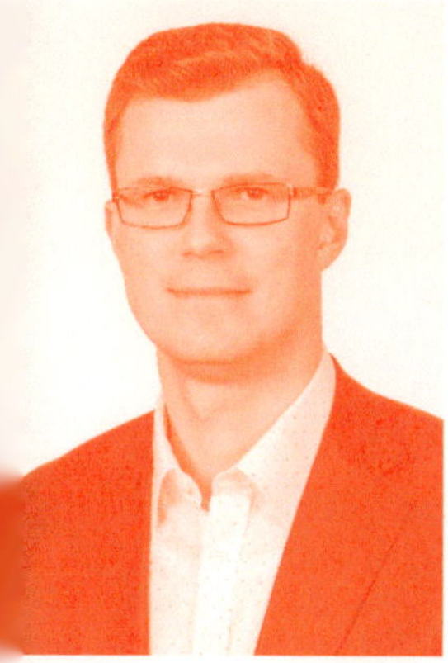
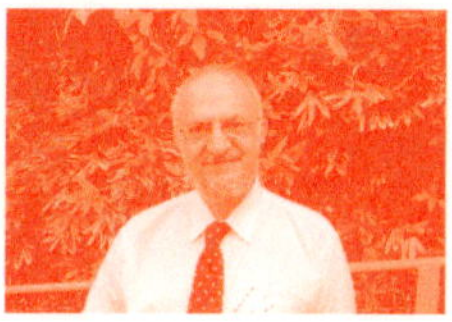
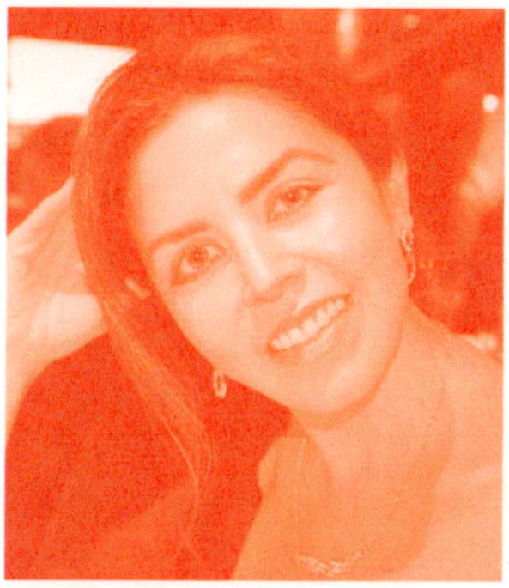

Supporting open minds since 2005

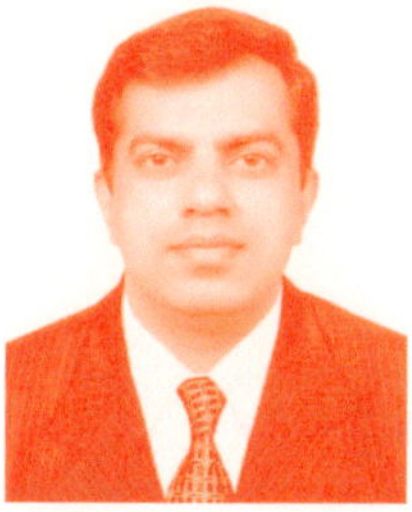
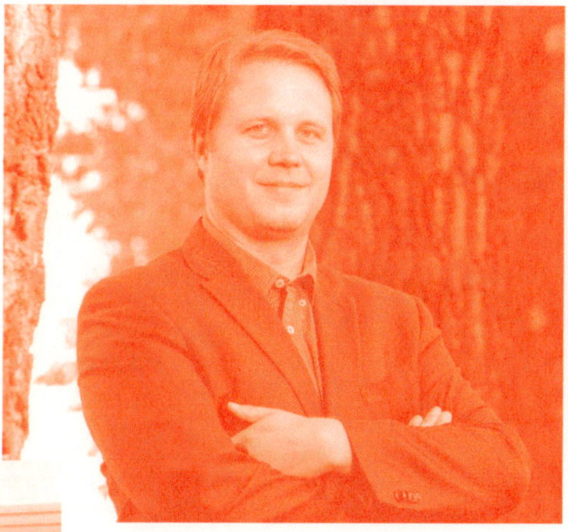
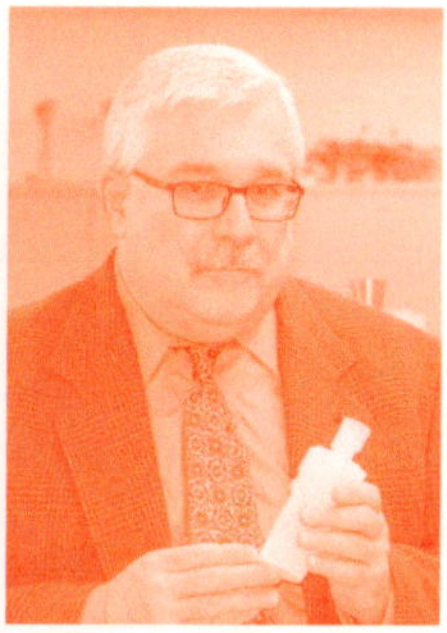
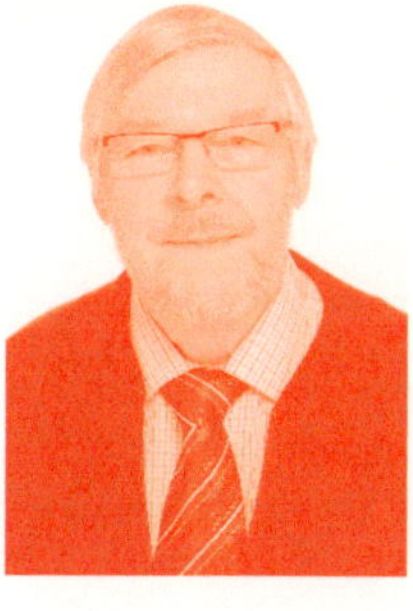
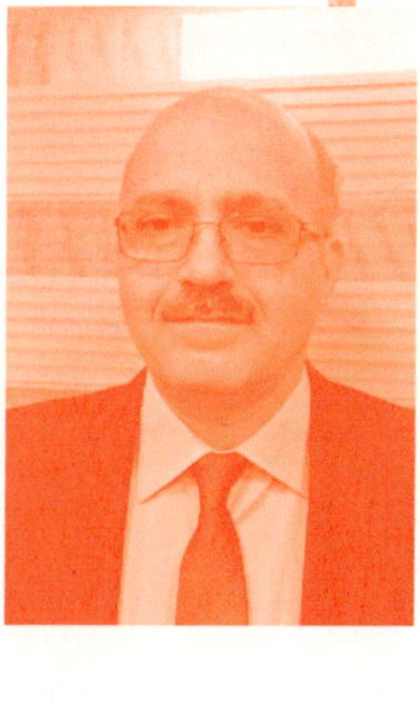
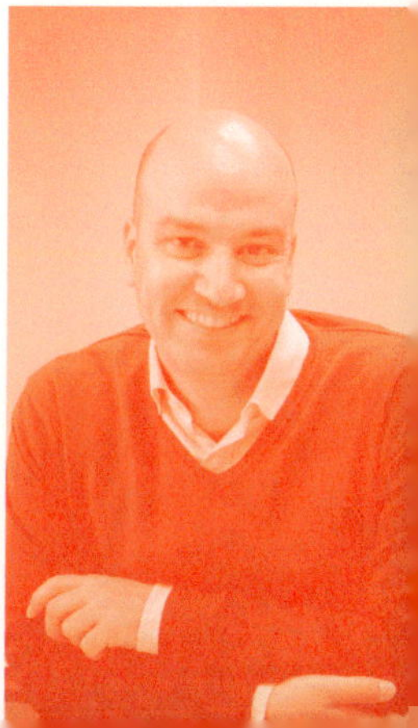
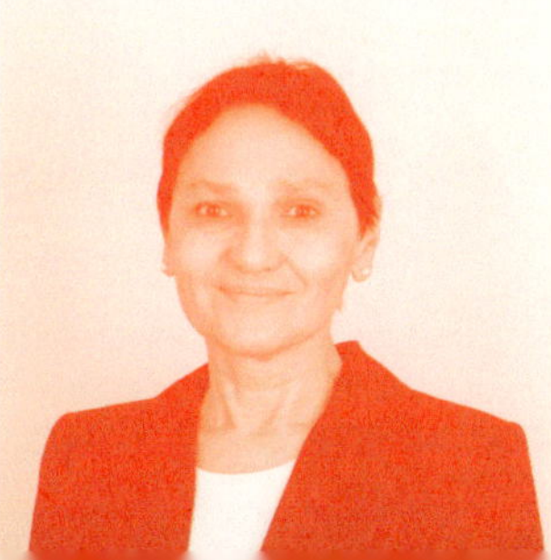

Antidepressants - Preclinical, Clinical and Translational Aspects
http://dx.doi.org/10.5772/intechopen.73911
Edited by Berend Olivier

Contributors
Gerard Marek, Mark Benvenga, Stephen Chaney, Jose Ontiveros, Laura Orio, Francisco Alén, Antonio Ballesta, Fernando Rodríguez De Fonseca, Raquel Gómez De Heras, Jocelien D.A. Olivier, Laura Staal, Olivier Berend, Tatiana Gudasheva

First published in London, United Kingdom, 2019 by IntechOpen
IntechOpen is the global imprint of INTECHOPEN LIMITED, registered in England and Wales, registration number: 11086078, 7th floor, 10 Lower Thames Street, London, EC3R 6AF, United Kingdom
Printed in Croatia

British Library Cataloguing-in-Publication Data
A catalogue record for this book is available from the British Library

Additional hard and PDF copies can be obtained from orders@intechopen.com

Antidepressants - Preclinical, Clinical and Translational Aspects
Edited by Berend Olivier
p. cm.
Print ISBN 978-1-78985-266-0
Online ISBN 978-1-78985-277-6
eBook (PDF) ISBN 978-1-78985-278-3

For EU product safety concerns:
IN TECH d.o.o., Prolaz Marije Krucifikse Kozulić 3, 51000 Rijeka, Croatia, info@intechopen.com or visit our website at intechopen.com.

Meet the editor

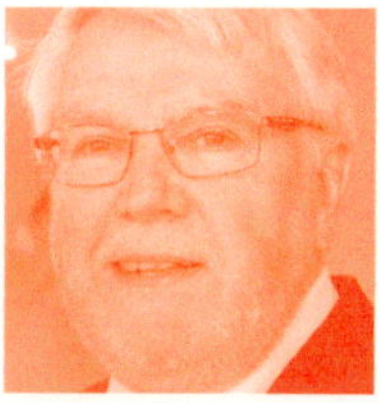

Berend Olivier obtained a PhD in Neurobiology from Groningen University, Netherlands. He worked for 22 years at Solvay Pharmaceuticals performing research and development on psychoactive drugs, including antidepressants, antipsychotics, anxiolytics and serenics, specifically aiming for reduction of pathological aggression. He was involved in research and development around fluvoxamine, an SSRI antidepressant, anxiolytic and anti-OCD medicine. In 1999–2001 he worked in New York to set up a biotech company, PsychoGenics Inc., developing animal psychiatric and neurological (genetic) models to find new psychoactive molecules. From 1992 to 2014 he was professor of CNS-Pharmacology at Utrecht University, Netherlands, performing fundamental research on animal models, brain mechanisms and pharmacology of psychiatric disorders. Dr. Olivier has published more than 600 scientific articles and book chapters.

Contents

Preface **XI**

Section 1
Introduction **1**

Chapter 1 **3**
Introductory Chapter: Antidepressants - Preclinical, Clinical and Translational Aspects
by Berend Olivier

Section 2
Clinical Studies **15**

Chapter 2 **17**
Rethinking the Use of Antidepressants to Treat Alcohol Use Disorders and Depression Comorbidity: The Role of Neurogenesis
by Antonio Ballesta, Francisco Alén, Fernando Rodríguez de Fonseca, Raquel Gómez de Heras and Laura Orio

Chapter 3 **37**
Resistant Depression
by Jose Alfonso Ontiveros

Section 3
Preclinical and Translational Studies **65**

Chapter 4 **67**
Influences of Maternal Vulnerability and Antidepressant Treatment during Pregnancy on the Developing Offspring
by Laura Staal and Jocelien DA Olivier

Chapter 5 **85**
Orexin 2 Receptor Antagonists from Prefrontal Cortical Circuitry to Rodent Behavioral Screens
by Gerard J. Marek, Stephen Chaney and Mark J. Benvenga

Chapter 6 103
The BDNF Loop 4 Dipeptide Mimetic Bis(*N*-monosuccinyl-L-seryl-L-lysine) hexamethylenediamide Is Active in a Depression Model in Mice after Acute Oral Administration
by Polina Povarnina, Yulia N. Firsova, Anna V. Tallerova, Armen G. Mezhlumyan, Sergey V. Kruglov, Tatiana A. Antipova, Tatiana A. Gudasheva and Sergey B. Seredenin

Preface

Major depression is a prevalent and severe brain disorder with a high disability burden, as measured by the Disability-Adjusted Life Years (DALY) metric. Antidepressants were discovered and developed starting in the 1950s and 1960s, however, all 'early' antidepressants were discovered by chance. Based on these early medications, intense research into new and better antidepressants was undertaken, leading to the development of selective serotonin reuptake inhibitors (SSRIs). SSRIs are a class of antidepressants popular in the late 1980s and 1990s that are still being used today. Although many new antidepressants with various mechanisms have been found and introduced, we still have not seen 'real' antidepressants, defined as drugs that 'repair' or 'improve' the depression-causing mechanism in the brains of depressed patients. Another worrying aspect is the limited efficacy of antidepressants; only around 50% of depressed patients respond to existing antidepressants and a considerable number does not respond at all (i.e., treatment-resistant depressed people). Another feature of present antidepressants is their slow onset of action. It takes weeks to moths before a depressed patient experiences improvement of symptoms (if a patient is a 'responder'). All antidepressants have side effects that may lead to cessation of treatment in an early phase before remission of depressive symptoms can occur. Although initially developed as therapy for depression, antidepressants are often also therapeutically active in other psychiatric disorders, like anxiety and obsessive-compulsive disorders or alcohol use disorders.

All these aspects of antidepressants are reflected in the various sections and chapters of this book. In Section 1, Berend Olivier (Chapter 1) gives an introductory sketch of preclinical, clinical and translational aspects of various antidepressants, including the development of potential new antidepressants with less side effects or faster onset of action and activity against treatment-resistant depression.

In Section 2 (Clinical Studies), Dr. Laura Orio et al. (Chapter 2) give an extensive overview of the use of antidepressants in alcohol use disorders and these disorders' comorbidity with depression. They particularly focus on the role of neurogenesis in the therapeutic effects of antidepressants by increasing hippocampal plasticity. They also discuss the possibility of implementing treatment during alcohol abstinence.

Dr. Ontiveros (Chapter 3) gives a thoughtful overview of treatment-resistant depression (TRD), a condition with serious medical and psychosocial complications. An exact definition of TRD is still subject of debate and much research still has to be done to find solutions. The chapter delves into this debate as well as discusses the many strategies that have been applied to help patients recover from severe depression.

In Section 3 (Preclinical and Translational Studies), Laura Staal and Jocelien Olivier (Chapter 4) discuss the problems associated with antidepressant treatment during pregnancy. Unfortunately, approximately 20% of pregnant women suffer from affective disorders. Treatment is beneficial for these women, but the long-term consequences of in utero treatment for their offspring is unclear. Untreated depression probably has adverse effects on offspring too, and this complicates the decisions on how to treat. The complex interactions – 'depression-mother-offspring-antidepressant' – are discussed in this intriguing contribution. The authors make clear that animal models are indispensable in making decisions on how to proceed.

The final two chapters deal with the search for new antidepressants. Dr. Marek et al. (Chapter 5) describe the theory of the potential of orexin2 receptor antagonists as antidepressants. In an animal model of depression, differential-reinforcement-of-low-rate 72-second schedule (DRL 72s), the orexin2 receptor antagonist LSN2424100 had antidepressant-like effects, comparable to the reference tricyclic antidepressant imipramine. Although clinical trials with orexin antagonists in depressed patients have not yet resulted in clear evidence for their antidepressant activity, this 'orexin' approach is a promising line of potential new antidepressants.

Dr. Tatiana Gudasheva et al. (Chapter 6) synthesize and further develop a low-molecular dipeptide BDNF-loop-4-mimetic, GSB-106, as a potential antidepressant, based on the role of BDNF in the pathophysiology of depression. By using an animal model that induces a depression-like state in mice via social defeat stress, GSB-106, like the tricyclic antidepressant amitriptyline, induced an antidepressant-like effect. Whether ligands that influence BDNF activity in the brain constitute putative new human antidepressants is a matter of future research.

This book nicely illustrates various aspects of the application of existing antidepressants and the drug discovery process, which is trying to identify and develop new and hopefully better antidepressants.

Professor Dr. Berend Olivier
Professor Emeritus Pharmacology of the Central Nervous System,
Faculty of Science,
Department of Psychopharmacology,
Utrecht University,
Utrecht, The Netherlands

Adjunct Professor
Department of Psychiatry,
Yale University School of Medicine,
New Haven, USA

Section 1

Introduction

Chapter 1

Introductory Chapter: Antidepressants - Preclinical, Clinical and Translational Aspects

Berend Olivier

1. Introduction

In 2011 two extensive studies were published about prevalence and associated disability, including the associated disease burden and financial costs, of brain diseases in Europe [1–3]. A shocking finding was that in a European population of more than 400 million people, approximately one-third suffered from a psychiatric or neurological disorder. In the psychiatric disorders, anxiety disorders had the highest 12-month prevalence (14%) and depression (7%), approximately 61.5 million people. The disability burden of psychiatric diseases including major depression is tremendous being defined in disability-adjusted life years (DALYs). In 2010, more than 26% of all cumulated disease burden in Europe was due to brain disorders; depression belongs to the top diseases with the highest DALYs. Major depression is a severe brain disorder associated with long-term disability and low quality of life. Suicide and suicidal attempts are highly associated with depression and have an enormous impact on relatives and society.

2. Antidepressants

Since the 1950s and 1960s of the last century, discovery and development of antidepressants have gradually emerged. Early antidepressants like imipramine and the irreversible monoamine oxidase inhibitors (MAOI) were discovered by serendipity. These "accidental" discoveries have led to intensive research and have led to a series of new antidepressants, like the tricyclic class (TCA, e.g., imipramine, nortriptyline, amitriptyline, and clomipramine) and a series of (both reversible and irreversible) MAOIs. These antidepressants, although still clinically available, are not anymore first-line medicines, mainly because of their sometimes severe side effects. The research in the 1960s and 1970s led to the insight that TCAs block monoamine transporters (reuptake carriers) for serotonin and noradrenaline to varying extent. Some TCAs are preferential serotonin transporter (SERT) blockers (clomipramine, amitriptyline), while others are preferential noradrenaline transporter (NET) blockers (desipramine, maprotiline) or mixed SERT/NET blockers (doxepin, imipramine). TCAs also block several neurotransmitter receptors, particularly muscarinic cholinergic, H_1 histaminergic, and α_1-adrenoceptors, which is mainly responsible for their (unwanted) side effects, including sedation, dry mouth, and constipation.

Based on the early, but overly simplistic hypothesis that low serotonin and/or noradrenalin levels/activity in the brain are associated (or even causative in) with depression, the development of selective serotonin reuptake inhibitors (SSRIs; fluoxetine, fluvoxamine, sertraline, paroxetine, citalopram, escitalopram) and selective noradrenaline reuptake inhibitors (NRIs; reboxetine, atomoxetine) and mixed 5-HT/NA reuptake blockers (SNRIs: venlafaxine, duloxetine) was enabled. Several other antidepressants have been developed (e.g., bupropion, mirtazapine, agomelatine, trazodone, nefazodone), with variable mechanisms of action. In general, SSRIs are the drugs of choice and first-line in the treatment of major depression [4]. The first SSRIs (zimeldine, fluvoxamine) were introduced in the early 1980s [5], and in the ensuing decade, several followed (fluoxetine, paroxetine, sertraline). Up to this moment, SSRIs still are first-line medication in MDD, but some breakthrough antidepressants are emerging (esketamine), whereas extensive and intensive research and development are ongoing [6].

3. Antidepressants: how good are they?

SSRIs like all antidepressants come with associated problems, viz., (1) side effects, (2) limited efficacy, and (3) slow onset of action.

3.1 Side effects

Major depressive disorder (MDD) typically comes in recurrent depressive episodes rather than a single episode. Antidepressant treatment requires to focus on both acute and maintenance aspects of MDD. The primary goal of the acute treatment phase (8–12 weeks) is to achieve symptomatic remission. In the acute phase, emerging side effects of the first-line treatment (often an SSRI) and the tolerance development of the patient strongly co-determine a positive antidepressant response to SSRIs or SNRIs. Main side effects (occurring in approximately 10–30% of patients) are nausea, dry mouth, sweating, sexual dysfunction, somnolence, nervousness, anxiety, dizziness, and insomnia [7]. If SSRI/SNRI treatment is not effective, MAO inhibitors or TCAs (as third-line treatments) may be used, although they come with additional and often more severe side effects. Second-line treatment includes novel antidepressants like vilazodone or vortioxetine or second-generation antidepressants like agomelatine, bupropion, or mirtazapine. All have their own side effect profile and are comparably effective antidepressant compared to SSRIs and others [8]. Lifetime major depression has high psychiatric comorbidity with anxiety disorders, substance use disorders, and impulse control disorders. Many depressed patients have medical (physical) comorbidities requiring pharmacotherapy, and this brings the risk of drug-drug interactions, often associated with cytochrome (CYP) P450 or P-glycoprotein-mediated effects. This may exacerbate side effects of drugs or interfere with the pharmacological action.

The most disturbing side effects of SSRIs and some TCAs (e.g., clomipramine) are those on sexual functioning like libido, orgasm, and arousal problems. In contrast to some other side effects that are prominent in the first phase of treatment, but often diminish upon drug continuation (like nausea and dizziness), sexual side effects do not disappear and are often causing drug discontinuation. MDD itself is already associated with 50–70% enhanced risk of sexual dysfunction (SD), and prescribing antidepressants with inherent effects on sexual behavior strongly enhances the risk for noncompliance or discontinued drug-taking [9]. Such a scenario can be avoided by prescribing (e.g., as second-line choice) antidepressants without (or less) sexual side effects (e.g., agomelatine, bupropion, vilazodone, or vortioxetine). Because depression occurs during all life phases, it is also common during pregnancy with an estimation of 20% of women that experience depressive symptoms during that time [10], whereas around 4–8% of pregnant women suffer from MDD. Depression of the mother impacts the fetus, e.g., by the enhanced cortisol levels in the mother which also pass the placenta. There is strong evidence that increased stress levels of the mother may lead to neurological and behavioral changes in the child which persists at least into adolescence (e.g., [11]). In the contribution of Staal and Olivier (Chapter 2), a review is given of the consequences of depression during pregnancy. Although the consequences for a child, adolescent, or adult that was in utero subject to a mother experiencing MDD are not yet completely clear, the first results point to a negative influence [12]. However, nowadays a considerable number (2–3%) of pregnant women with MDD are treated with antidepressants, mostly with SSRIs. SSRIs cross the placenta and reach the fetus, including the central nervous system. Because serotonin plays a key role in embryonic development as a neurotrophic factor, disturbances in its level might lead to (permanent) changes in the offspring [13–15]. Chapter 2 summarizes the state of the art of the interaction between untreated or SSRI-treated mothers with severe depression. It is not yet clear whether SSRI treatment or not is preferable for depression in pregnant women.

3.2 Limited efficacy

Antidepressants have limited efficacy in relieving depressive symptoms in MDD patients. It is estimated that approximately 50% of depressed patients are adequately treated by the available interventions, including pharmacotherapy [16]. Most patients receiving pharmacotherapy fail to achieve and sustain remission, eventually not leading to functional recovery. The majority of patients starting an antidepressant require several subsequent and different antidepressants or adjunctive therapy (either pharmacological or cognitive behavioral therapy). There is evidence that if a chosen treatment strategy (a certain antidepressant, often an SSRI) results in symptomatic improvement within the first weeks, full remission is likely, but the reverse is also true: lack of early improvement predicts a high chance on non-remittance [17]. After failure of a number of (adequately dosed) antidepressants of different classes (SSRI, TCA, MAOI), and augmentation with various drugs (e.g., antipsychotics) and other strategies (e.g., cognitive behavioral therapy), patients are considered treatment-resistant. Treatment-resistant depression (TRD) is defined as the failure to respond to one or more standard antidepressant treatment trials of adequate dosing and duration [18, 19]. TRD is a big challenge to treat. Although depression is diagnosed as a single entity, MDD [20] is an extremely heterogeneous disease [21] with regard to symptoms, etiologies, and pathophysiologies, with some moderately heritable background [22] and a high susceptibility to adverse life events [23]. TRD reflects a complex, heterogeneous state, probably with multiple causal underlying mechanisms. It is not clear how and where TRD patients differ from non-TRD patients, although early life stress seems to facilitate treatment resistance [24]. Research is clearly needed to establish the pathophysiology of TRD, the complex mechanisms involved, and the heterogeneity of the TRD patient. Unfortunately, depression is presently not a high priority for pharmaceutical companies, due to recent failures in antidepressant discovery and lack of understanding of the mechanisms involved and the consequent lack of available targets. Akil et al. [21] argue a need of a fundamental approach in the search for new and effective treatments for TRD. They propose to identify dysfunctional brain circuitry in animal models of depression, looking at changes in associated gene expression. Combination of animal research with human genetic and imaging studies must generate circuits and molecules that are both altered in the animal models of TRD and also in selected patient populations. Such translational and highly integrated research may lead to new targets for specific anti-TRD medication.

In Chapter 3 Marek and colleagues describe the research on orexin 2 receptor antagonists as putative new antidepressants. Orexin, a hypothalamic neuropeptide, is known for its involvement in sleep-wake cycling of all mammals, including man. Orexin 2 receptor antagonists produce antidepressant activity in animal tests sensitive for antidepressant activity, including the DRL-72 sec schedule of reinforcement, an advanced screen for antidepressants [25]. Both positive and negative preliminary human data are present on orexin 2 receptor antagonists in depression, but further studies are needed to answer whether this approach might lead to new antidepressants or may be also effective in treatment-resistant depression.

3.3 Slow onset of action

The current most widely prescribed antidepressants, SSRIs and SNRIs, but also TCAs and MAOIs and other antidepressants, have no acute onset of action but work (gradually) over a period of weeks to months. It is still largely unknown what underlying CNS mechanisms are involved in the slow onset of action of antidepressants. In the case of serotonergic antidepressants (SSRIs, SNRIs), a complex interaction between various 5-HT auto- and heteroreceptors as modulators of the SSRI-induced chronic increase in CNS serotonin plays a role [26]. Acute administration of SSRIs Inhibits somatodendritic 5-HT_{1A} autoreceptors leading to inhibition of firing activity of serotonergic neurons and consequently dampened release of 5-HT in the forebrain, which, in some not yet understood way, contributes to the slow onset of action of SSRIs [27]. Desensitization of 5-HT_{1A} autoreceptors after long-term administration might overcome the decrease in 5-HT release and subsequently would lead to high serotonin release [27]. Combining an SSRI and 5-HT_{1A}-receptor antagonist might create a fast onset of action mechanism for antidepressant activity. The lack of availability of clinically approved selective 5-HT_{1A} receptor antagonists led to studies using the mixed β-adrenoceptor/5-HT_{1A} receptor antagonist pindolol together with various SSRIs in MDD patients [28]. In a placebo-controlled study, pindolol increased the antidepressant efficacy of fluoxetine, although no significant improvement in onset of action of the combination was found [29]. Pindolol is probably not the best tool to perform this kind of "onset of action" studies (pindolol is a relatively weak and not a full 5-HT_{1A} receptor antagonist, and its beta-blocking activities induce side effects), but a study with a selective 5-HT_{1A}-receptor antagonist did not find any difference either. It was postulated [30, 31] that two new multi-target antidepressants, vilazodone (SSRI+ partial 5-HT_{1A} receptor agonist) and vortioxetine (SSRI+5-$HT_{1A,1B,1D,7}$ receptor agonist and 5-HT_3 receptor antagonist), might have an advantage over existing drugs in terms of efficacy and onset of antidepressant action, although clinical data thus far have not shown evidence for improving the onset of action [32, 33]. It is evident that antidepressants that primarily act via monoaminergic neurotransmission all share the slow onset of action principle, and new molecules stemming from this "classical" approach will not deliver fast onset of action compounds.

The finding that one single dose of intravenous ketamine produced rapid and sustained antidepressant effects in depressed patients led to a new and exciting opening in this field [34]. Ketamine, an NMDA receptor antagonist and dissociative anesthetic, produces at low doses mild dissociative and psychotomimetic effects but also exerted rather unexpected antidepressant effects. One single dose of ketamine (0.5 mg/kg, intravenously by slow infusion) induced a rapid antidepressant effect (within hours) that lasted for 7 days [35]. Later studies have confirmed the fast antidepressant onset, even in TRD patients [6]. However, notwithstanding the apparent breakthrough in fast treatment of depression, the side effects of ketamine are still troublesome for general use. Recently (March 2019) a nasal preparation of the (S)-enantiomer (esketamine) received FDA approval after successful phase 3 trials. Moreover, new approaches for fast-onset and effective antidepressants via modulation of the glutamatergic-NMDA system are now subject of intense research efforts [6, 36]. One may expect a new range of novel antidepressants with as main attribute a fast onset of action. Whether these new molecules have a higher efficacy (>50% of responding patients) or accordingly lead to less treatment resistance has to be awaited. Moreover, the side effect profile is likely quite different from the classical "monoaminergic" antidepressants. Only large number of well-treated patients will unravel the impact of these side effects. If only the onset of action is improved, the acceptance of such a new antidepressant will strongly depend on its side effect and safety profile.

One of the big items in the research and discovery of new and innovative antidepressants is the availability of animal models that are able to measure "onset of action," "efficacy," and "side effects" [37]. Onset of antidepressant action in an animal model is quite difficult to assess. Most animal depression tests are acute, in that they respond immediately to a dose of a certain antidepressant, e.g., forced swim test, tail suspension test, or DRL-72 sec paradigm. Animal depression models that do not respond acutely but only after chronic treatment of the classic antidepressants are rather scarce, although indispensable in the onset of action discovery. One of such models is the olfactory bulbectomized (OBX) rat [37, 38]. OBX leads to stable and lasting changes in behavior after removing the olfactory bulbs [39]. OBX leads within days after ablation to permanent changes in activity, basal body temperature, heart rate and heart rate variability, and stress responsivity [39]. Increased locomotor activity in an open field is an often used simple parameter to measure the effects of antidepressants [38]. In an extensive review on available animal models, olfactory bulbectomy in rodents is considered superior to other animal models to detect onset of action of antidepressants [37], with a high sensitivity, specificity, and reliability and moderate ease to use the model. The model generated also the possibility to study effects of antidepressant treatment after cessation of treatment [40]. Chronic (14-day) treatment of imipramine (20 mg/kg) or escitalopram (5 and 10 mg/kg) in OBX and sham-operated rats led to reduction of the hyperactivity in an open field by imipramine and escitalopram of the OBX rats, without effects in the control rats. This reduction in hyperactivity of OBX rats induced by chronic administration of antidepressants remained after cessation of treatment and lasted for 10 weeks after imipramine and 6 weeks after escitalopram cessation [40]. We concluded that the OBX-induced changes in the brain state (neuroplasticity) are probably attenuated by chronic antidepressant administration and that these changes are only slowly returning to the previous OBX state. Pramipexole, a dopamine D3/D2 receptor agonist, used to treat Parkinson patients with additional antidepressant activity [41], indeed exerted antidepressant activity in the OBX model [42]. Pramipexole is also a psychostimulant and induces at higher doses enhanced locomotion itself, thereby interfering with the already enhanced activity of OBX rats. Remarkably, 1 week after cessation of treatment, pramipexole-treated OBX animals still were not hyperactive, similar to imipramine, thereby suggesting that antidepressant effects of drugs can be detected in the OBX model by using this post-cessation antidepressant-like effect [42]. Unpublished studies [43] found that 3- and 7-day treatment with imipramine (10 mg/kg/day) normalized OBX-induced hyperactivity in the open field. One week after cessation of imipramine treatment, hyperactivity returned, suggesting that longer periods of treatment (14 days) are at least needed to lead to changes in brain neuroplasticity underlying the suppression of OBX-induced behavioral changes. In a complicated experimental design, ketamine (10 mg/kg, IP) was given to OBX and control rats 24 hours before testing in an open field but appeared ineffective [44]. The experimental design did not give a clear cue about the onset of action of antidepressant activity of ketamine, and more directed research into this avenue has to be initiated. Pandey et al. [45] found that

14-day but not 7-day treatment with ketamine (1 mg/kg/day) reduced hyperactivity induced by olfactory bulbectomy, although combination of escitalopram (10 mg/kg/day) and ketamine (1 mg/kg/day) reduced hyperactivity at both 7 and 14 days. This may be an indication that ketamine in combination with an SSRI may speed up the onset of antidepressant action.

Recently the FDA has approved esketamine as a nasal spray for adjunctive therapy in treatment-resistant depression [46]. Esketamine is indicated for depressed patients that did not respond to at least two oral antidepressant monotherapies. It has to be given together with a newly initiated oral antidepressant under strict supervision of certified medical professionals, because of the potential serious adverse effects of esketamine. The launch of a successful potential anti-TRD medication might be a breakthrough in the treatment of depression.

4. Other applications for antidepressants

Apart from treatment of depression, antidepressants and particularly SSRIs and SNRIs are also widely used for treatment of various anxiety disorders, obsessive compulsive disorders, gambling disorders, posttraumatic stress disorder, and various other psychiatric disorders, including alcohol use disorder.

In obsessive compulsive disorder, SSRIs are partially effective, but in general higher doses are needed, and onset of action (6–8 weeks) is slower than in depression. Because comorbidity of depression and anxiety is very high, it appeared that SSRIs could be used as a rational therapy for both disorders, although the disadvantages of SSRIs in depression (side effects, onset of action, partial efficacy) are comparable in anxiety disorder treatment. In Chapter 4, Ballesta and coworkers review and discuss the role of antidepressants in alcohol use disorder (AUD). Because a strong relationship exists between major depression and AUD, the authors investigated the potential role of hippocampal plasticity and neurogenesis in both disorders. By integrating the knowledge of plasticity changes in the hippocampus and its role in both disorders, the authors try to implement shared mechanisms. It is clear that considerable research efforts, both preclinical and clinical, are needed to advance our possibilities to better treat both depression and alcohol use disorder.

5. Conclusion

The emergence of effective antidepressants in the 1960s and 1970s of the last century has led to an explosion of new and often unexpected new discoveries and clinical applications. The development of SSRIs after the serendipitous detection of the first tricyclic antidepressants has revolutionized the treatment of major depression but has also led to new treatments of various anxiety disorders, obsessive compulsive disorder, and various other psychiatric conditions.

Drug treatment always leads to side effects that can be quite cumbersome and often lead to drug discontinuation. Treatment resistance (TRD) is frequently occurring in major depression, and a substantial part of depressed patients (about 30%) does not respond to any treatment. Recent developments (esketamine) promise new approaches in the treatment of TRD although side effects remain a big obstacle.

Research into new and better antidepressants remains urgent but depends primarily on better understanding of the brain mechanisms involved in normal "mood" processing and understanding what is wrong in "depressed" brains. Animal models with high predictive and construct validity are urgently needed to help to discover these (dys)functional mechanisms and deliver new targets for better antidepressants.

Author details

Berend Olivier[1,2]

1 Department of Psychopharmacology, Utrecht Institute for Pharmaceutical Sciences, Utrecht University, Utrecht, The Netherlands

2 Department of Psychiatry, Yale University School of Medicine, New Haven, USA

*Address all correspondence to: b.olivier@uu.nl

References

[1] Wittchen HU, Jacobi F, Rehm J, Gustavsson A, Svensson M, Jönsson B, et al. The size and burden of mental disorders and other disorders of the brain in Europe 2010. European Neuropsychopharmacology. 2011;**21**:655-679

[2] Gustavsson A, Svensson M, Jacobi F, Allgulander C, Alonso J, Berghi E, et al. Cost of disorders of the brain in Europe 2010. European Neuropsychopharmacology. 2011;**21**:717-778

[3] Nutt DJ. The full cost and burden of disorders of the brain in Europe exposed for the first time. European Neuropsychopharmacology. 2011;**21**:715-717

[4] Balon R. Modifications of the serotonin system by antidepressant treatments: Implications for the therapeutic response in major depression. The American Journal of Psychiatry. 2006;**163**:1504-1509

[5] Olivier B. Serotonin: A never-ending story. European Journal of Pharmacology. 2015;**753**:2-18

[6] Duman RS, Shinohara R, Fogaça MV, Hare B. Neurobiology of rapid-acting antidepressants: Convergent effects on GluA1-synaptic function. Molecular Psychiatry. 2019. DOI: 10.1038/s41380-019-0400-x

[7] Kennedy SH, Lam RW, McIntyre RS, Tourjman SV, Bhat V, Blier P, et al. CANMAT depression work group. Canadian network for mood and anxiety treatments (CANMAT) 2016 clinical guidelines for the management of adults with major depressive disorder: Section 3. Pharmacological treatments. Canadian Journal of Psychiatry. 2016;**61**(9):540-560. DOI: 10.1177/0706743716659417.

[8] Rush AJ, Trivedi MH, Wisniewski SR, Nierenberg AA, Stewart JW, Warden D, et al. Acute and longer-term outcomes in depressed outpatients requiring one or several treatment steps: A STAR*D report. The American Journal of Psychiatry. 2006;**163**(11):1905-1917

[9] Chokka PR, Hankey JR. Assessment and management of sexual dysfunction in the context of depression. Therapeutic Advances in Psychopharmacology. 2018;**8**(1):13-23

[10] Ryan D, Milis L, Misri N. Depression during pregnancy. Canadian Family Physician. 2005;**51**:1087-1093

[11] Hutchison SM, Mâsse LC, Brain U, Oberlander TF. A 6-year longitudinal study: Are maternal depressive symptoms and selective serotonin reuptake inhibitor (SSRI) antidepressant treatment during pregnancy associated with everyday measures of executive function in young children? Early Human Development. 2019;**128**:21-26. DOI: 10.1016/j.earlhumdev.2018.10.009

[12] Houwing DJ, Staal L, Swart JM, Ramsteijn AS, Wöhr M, de Boer SF, et al. Subjecting dams to early life stress and perinatal fluoxetine treatment differentially alters social behavior in young and adult rat offspring. Frontiers in Neuroscience. 2019;**13**:229. DOI: 10.3389/fnins.2019.00229

[13] Weissman MM. Postpartum depression and its long-term impact on children: Many new questions. JAMA Psychiatry. 2018;**75**(3):227-228. DOI: 10.1001/jamapsychiatry.2017.4265

[14] Malm H, Brown AS, Gissler M, Gyllenberg D, Hinkka-Yli-Salomäki S, McKeague IW, et al. Gestational exposure to selective serotonin reuptake inhibitors and offspring psychiatric

disorders: A National Register-Based Study. Journal of the American Academy of Child and Adolescent Psychiatry. 2016;**55**(5):359-366. DOI: 10.1016/j.jaac.2016.02.013

[15] Gaspar P, Cases O, Maroteaux L. The developmental role of serotonin: News from mouse molecular genetics. Nature Reviews Neuroscience. 2003;**4**:1002-1012

[16] McIntyre RS, Filteau MJ, Martin L, Patry S, Carvalho A, Cha DS, et al. Treatment-resistant depression: Definitions, review of the evidence, and algorithmic approach. Journal of Affective Disorders. 2014;**156**:1-7. DOI: 10.1016/j.jad.2013.10.043

[17] Kudlow PA, Cha DS, McIntyre RS. Predicting treatment response in major depressive disorder: The impact of early symptomatic improvement. Canadian Journal of Psychiatry. 2012;**57**(12):782-788

[18] Papakostas GI, Ionescu DF. Towards new mechanisms: An update on therapeutics for treatment-resistant major depressive disorder. Molecular Psychiatry. 2015;**20**(10):1142-1150. DOI: 10.1038/mp.2015.92

[19] Fava M. Diagnosis and definition of treatment-resistant depression. Biological Psychiatry. 2003;**53**(8):649-659

[20] DSM5. American Psychiatric Association Diagnostic and Statistical Manual of Mental Disorders. 5th ed. Arlington, VA: American Psychiatric Association; 2013

[21] Akil H, Gordon J, Hen R, Javitch J, Mayberg H, McEwen B, et al. Treatment resistant depression: A multi-scale, systems biology approach. Neuroscience and Biobehavioral Reviews. 2018;**84**:272-288. DOI: 10.1016/j.neubiorev.2017.08.019

[22] Geschwind DH, Flint J. Genetics and genomics of psychiatric disease. Science. 2015;**349**(6255):1489-1494. DOI: 10.1126/science.aaa8954

[23] Otte C, Gold SM, Penninx BW, Pariante CM, Etkin A, Fava M, et al. Major depressive disorder. Nature Reviews Disease Primers. 2016;**2**:16065. DOI: 10.1038/nrdp.2016.65

[24] Williams LM. Precision psychiatry: A neural circuit taxonomy for depression and anxiety. Lancet Psychiatry. 2016;**3**(5):472-480. DOI: 10.1016/S2215-0366(15)00579-9

[25] O'Donnell JM, Marek GJ, Seiden LS. Antidepressant effects assessed using behavior maintained under a differential-reinforcement-of-low-rate (DRL) operant schedule. Neuroscience and Biobehavioral Reviews. 2005;**29**(4-5):785-798

[26] Nautiyal KM, Hen R. Serotonin receptors in depression: From A to B. F1000Res. 2017;**6**:123. DOI: 10.12688/f1000research.9736.1. eCollection 2017

[27] Artigas F, Romero L, de Montigny C, Blier P. Acceleration of the effect of selected antidepressant drugs in major depression by 5-HT1A antagonists. Trends in Neurosciences. 1996;**19**(9):378-383

[28] Artigas F, Schenker E, Celada P, Spedding M, Lladó-Pelfort L, Jurado N, et al. Defining the brain circuits involved in psychiatric disorders: IMI-NEWMEDS. Nature Reviews Drug Discovery. 2017;**16**(1):1-2. DOI: 10.1038/nrd.2016.205

[29] Pérez V, Gilaberte I, Faries D, Alvarez E, Artigas F. Randomised, double-blind, placebo-controlled trial of Pindolol in combination with fluoxetine antidepressant treatment. Lancet. 1997;**349**:1594-1597

[30] Scorza MC, Lladó-Pelfort L, Oller S, Cortés R, Puigdemont D, Portella MJ, et al. Preclinical and clinical characterization of the selective 5-HT(1A) receptor antagonist DU-125530 for antidepressant treatment. British Journal of Pharmacology. 2012;**167**(5):1021-1034. DOI: 10.1111/j.1476-5381.2011.01770.x

[31] Artigas F, Bortolozzi A, Celada P. Can we increase speed and efficacy of antidepressant treatments? Part I: General aspects and monoamine-based strategies. European Neuropsychopharmacology. 2018;**28**(4):445-456. DOI: 10.1016/j.euroneuro.2017.10.032

[32] Stuivenga M, Giltay EJ, Cools O, Roosens L, Neels H, Sabbe B. Evaluation of vilazodone for the treatment of depressive and anxiety disorders. Expert Opinion on Pharmacotherapy. 2019;**20**(3):251-260. DOI: 10.1080/14656566.2018.1549542

[33] Gonda X, Sharma SR, Tarazi FI. Vortioxetine: A novel antidepressant for the treatment of major depressive disorder. Expert Opinion on Drug Discovery. 2019;**14**(1):81-89. DOI: 10.1080/17460441.2019.1546691

[34] Berman RM, Cappiello A, Anand A, Oren DA, Heninger GR, Charney DS, et al. Antidepressant effects of ketamine in depressed patients. Biological Psychiatry. 2000;**47**(4):351-354

[35] Zarate CA Jr, Singh JB, Carlson PJ, Brutsche NE, Ameli R, Luckenbaugh DA, et al. A randomized trial of an N-methyl-D-aspartate antagonist in treatment-resistant major depression. Archives of General Psychiatry. 2006;**63**(8):856-864

[36] Pham TH, Gardier AM. Fast-acting antidepressant activity of ketamine: Highlights on brain serotonin, glutamate, and GABA neurotransmission in preclinical studies. Pharmacology & Therapeutics. 2019;(pii):S0163-7258(19)30040-3. DOI: 10.1016/j.pharmthera.2019.02.017

[37] Ramaker MJ, Dulawa SC. Identifying fast-onset antidepressants using rodent models. Molecular Psychiatry. 2017;**22**(5):656-665. DOI: 10.1038/mp.2017.36

[38] Song C, Leonard BE. The olfactory bulbectomised rat as a model of depression. Neuroscience and Biobehavioral Reviews. 2005;**29**(4-5):627-647

[39] Vinkers CH, Breuer ME, Westphal KGC, Korte SM, Oosting RS, Olivier B, et al. Olfactory bulbectomy induces rapid and stable changes in basal and stress-induced locomotor activity, heart rate and body temperature responses in the home cage. Neuroscience. 2009;**159**:39-46

[40] Breuer ME, Groenink L, Oosting RS, Westenberg HGM, Olivier B. Long-term behavioral changes after cessation of chronic anti-depressant treatment in olfactory bulbectomized rats. Biological Psychiatry. 2007;**61**:990-995

[41] Barone P, Scarzella L, Marconi R, Antonini A, Morgante L, Bracco F, et al. Depression/Parkinson Italian study group. Pramipexole versus sertraline in the treatment of depression in Parkinson's disease: A national multicenter parallel-group randomized study. Journal of Neurology. 2006;**253**(5):601-607

[42] Breuer ME, Groenink L, Oosting RS, Buerger E, Korte SM, Ferger B, et al. Antidepressant effects of pramipexole, a dopamine D3/D2 receptor agonist in olfactory bulbectomized rats. European Journal of Pharmacology. 2009;**616**:134-140

[43] Breuer ME. Depression's next top model: Pharmacology of olfactory bulbectomy-induced behaviors [Ph.D. thesis]. Utrecht; 2009. pp. 1-185

[44] Holubova K, Kleteckova L, Skurlova M, Ricny J, Stuchlik A, Vales K. Rapamycin blocks the antidepressant effect of ketamine in task-dependent manner. Psychopharmacology. 2016;**233**(11):2077-2097. DOI: 10.1007/s00213-016-4256-3

[45] Pandey DK, Bhatt S, Jindal A, Gautam B. Effect of combination of ketanserin and escitalopram on behavioral anomalies after olfactory bulbectomy: Prediction of quick onset of antidepressant action. Indian Journal of Pharmacology. 2014;**46**(6):639-643. DOI: 10.4103/0253-7613.144935

[46] Sancar F. New therapy for treatment-resistant depression. Journal of the American Medical Association. 2019;**321**(15):1449. DOI: 10.1001/jama.2019.3596

Section 2

Clinical Studies

Chapter 2

Rethinking the Use of Antidepressants to Treat Alcohol Use Disorders and Depression Comorbidity: The Role of Neurogenesis

Antonio Ballesta, Francisco Alén, Fernando Rodríguez de Fonseca, Raquel Gómez de Heras and Laura Orio

Abstract

Patients with alcohol use disorders (AUDs) are frequently treated with antidepressant drugs (ADs), but clinical evidence of their efficacy is contradictory. Considering that ADs are thought to produce their therapeutic effects partially by increasing hippocampal plasticity and neurogenesis (HN), and that both AUDs and depression share a potential for the disruption of these neuroplastic processes, one could reasonably wonder whether the poor efficacy of AD treatment could be explained by the inability of these drugs to exert their proper action in patients suffering from AUD or depression. In order to further clarify this question, this chapter aims to examine available data regarding the effect of ADs on behavioral and HN alterations related to alcohol abstinence, as a key period in which the treatment would be implemented and in which their potential effects on alcohol-related problems remain under controversy.

Keywords: alcohol use disorders (AUDs), antidepressants (ADs), hippocampal neurogenesis (HN), depression, comorbidity, alcohol withdrawal

1. Introduction

AUD is a chronic relapsing brain disease characterized by the presence of various symptoms, such as physically hazardous alcohol drinking, tolerance, withdrawal, or craving related to alcohol consumption, whereas MD is a psychiatric disorder characterized by low mood, anhedonia, insomnia, low motivation, apathy, and feelings of guilt, among other symptoms [1]. Epidemiological studies have shown a strong relationship between alcohol use disorders (AUDs) and depression. Indeed, the prevalence of current or lifetime alcohol problems in depression is estimated around 16% and 30%, respectively [2].

Adult hippocampal neurogenesis (HN) is a complex multistep process by which neural progenitor cells (NPCs) divide throughout life and give rise to new functional neurons in restricted regions of the adult mammalian brain (**Figure 1**, and also described in [3]). The dentate gyrus of the hippocampus is one of the brain areas that respond to stimuli through multiple mechanisms that allow the proliferation,

IntechOpen

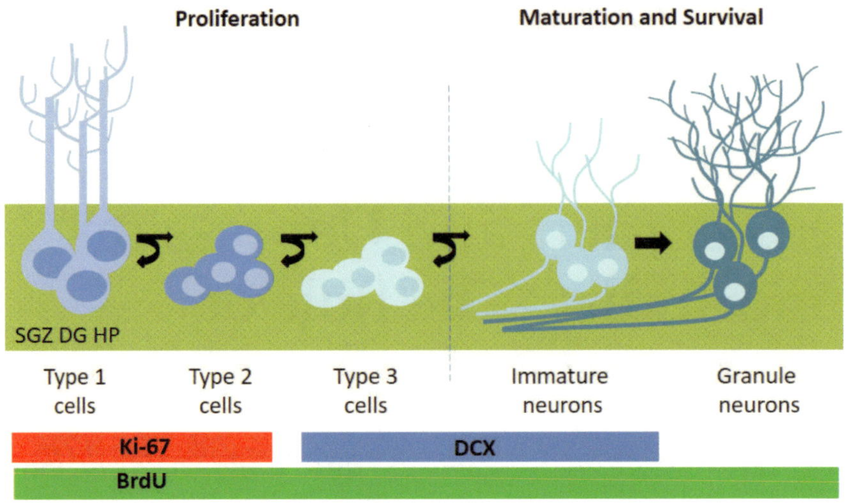

Figure 1.
Schematic representation of the stages of adult hippocampal neurogenesis in the subgranular zone of the dentate gyrus and the main immunolabeling techniques used in the cited studies.

maturation, and integration of new generated neurons in this structure, an event that appears to regulate and improve impaired cognition and mood in various disorders [4]. Both AUDs and depression have shown to compromise HN processes [5, 6]. The HN theory of depression sustains that depression results from impaired adult HN, and, therefore, its restoration leads to recovery [7]. Direct causality of HN alterations in the pathogenesis of depression seems unlikely [8], but the clinical relevance of hippocampal newly generated neurons in depression continues to be the object of study [9]. In addition, HN and plasticity processes have been proposed as a possible common neurobiological mechanism underlying alcohol withdrawal and depression [10]. In fact, HN has been proposed to significantly contribute to alcoholic pathology, although the mechanisms of alcohol-induced alterations in HN are not completely understood [6]. In this sense, there is strong evidence in animal models that alcoholic neuropathology is at least partially due to an attenuation of adult HN induced by intoxication, a state that could be reversed by spontaneous reactive HN processes during abstinence [11]. In this regard, authors have proposed that while suppression of hippocampal neurogenic proliferation appears to be a factor of comorbid vulnerability, enhancing HN into the neural circuits affected by drug may contribute to recovery [12, 13].

Antidepressants (ADs), mainly selective serotonin reuptake inhibitors (SSRIs) and tricyclic antidepressants (TCAs), are the primary pharmacological treatment indicated for depression-diagnosed patients [14]. Concurrently, evidence of monoamine alterations in AUDs has encouraged the investigation of drugs that act on the serotonin system to treat alcohol abuse [15]. Only a few drugs with clear evidence but modest effects are approved for treatment of AUDs, as naltrexone and acamprosate, although given certain clinical circumstances, substance use disorders may require specific treatment; thus, off-label medications like ADs are also frequently prescribed, mainly in AUD depressed patients [16]. At first, the monoamine theory of depression is based on the fact that brain monoamine systems appear to regulate mood and traditional ADs, such as SSRI, and selectively increase monoamine signaling in neural pathways related to mood regulation [17]. Later, at the beginning of the century, different results supported the hypothesis that ADs might affect mood by increasing adult HN [18]. At the same time, numerous studies have led to propose that ADs can influence HN by serotonin modulation and that HN may be related to AD effects (reviewed in [19]). In agreement, postmortem studies have reported that ADs augment NPC numbers [20, 21] and restore mature hippocampal neural population and dentate gyrus volume of depressed patients [22, 23]. These human data reflect the neurogenic potential of ADs previously reported in animals [24]. In this respect, animal studies have led to suggest that, while not causally involved in the onset of depression, HN has been related to the ability of chronic monoaminergic ADs to achieve recovery [8]. Recent studies have reopened the debate about the functional implication of adult HN in humans (see [25]), highlighting the need to further study the generation of new neurons in the adult human hippocampus. This also implies to characterize the role of HN in depression and AUDs [4, 6] and the extent to which it participates in recovery in the treatment with ADs [26].

2. Alcohol use disorders and depression

Data from AUD patients have led to the proposal that the effective components of withdrawal, such as dysphoria and depressed mood, create a motivational drive that leads to compulsive ethanol drinking behavior even after long periods of abstinence [27]. Subsequent findings promoted the hypothesis that drugs of abuse elicit pronounced euphoria followed by a negative emotional state that can disrupt homeostasis, considered key to the etiology and maintenance of the pathophysiology of addiction [28].

2.1 Clinical and preclinical evidence of AUD contribution to depressive symptomatology

Authors have considered whether there may be a causal relationship between AUDs and depression and whether one of the disorders can lead to the appearance of the other. Thus, numerous studies reveal ample evidence of the risk of depression resulting from AUDs [29]. Moreover, problematic patterns of alcohol consumption are related to depressive symptomatology, both in adult and adolescent populations [30, 31]. In an attempt to simplify the complexities of the relation between AUDs and depression, a classification of depression as primary or secondary according to whether it developed before or after the onset of the AUD was proposed. The term independent (ID) was used for a depression that began before the onset of alcohol dependence or during sustained (at least 4 weeks) abstinence, while depressive syndromes occurring only during a period of active alcohol dependence were labeled as substance-induced (SID) [32]. However, some of the depressive symptoms classified as ID could actually be substance-induced, as SID appears not to be a stable diagnosis, with about one quarter of patients initially labeled with SID meeting criteria for ID within the next 12 months [33]. Thus, SID would be considered a self-limiting condition that would tend to remit with abstinence, while ID would require specific depression treatment [32]. After receiving treatment for alcohol consumption, those with SID would show better depression outcomes and reduce their drinking more than those with ID [32]. Also, and further supporting a causal role of alcohol consumption in depression, reducing its consumption would improve the outcomes for both types of depression [34]. In the same sense, some authors have proposed that reducing hazardous drinking can improve depressive symptoms, but continued hazardous use slows recovery for psychiatric patients [35].

2.2 Preclinical evidence of the contribution of alcohol to depressive-like behavior

Animal studies might overcome the limitations of the clinical studies, allowing to obtain not only correlative information but also contributing data that would allow a larger approach to the possible underlying causes in the relation of the AUD and depression. Several preclinical studies have assessed behavioral alterations during acute withdrawal and/or protracted abstinence in different animal models of alcohol abuse [36–47]. Studies used rodents as experimental animals, and the majority used the AUD model of chronic intermittent ethanol (CIE) vapor exposure. Behavioral analysis was carried out from a few hours (less than 24 hours) to several days or weeks after the last alcohol consumption, using the forced swimming test (FST) the most frequently used paradigm for this purpose. FST allows detecting responses toward an inescapable stress in animals based on the measurement of the time they remain immobile rather than displaying active strategies, akin to responses that would be impaired in depression. This response has been commonly described in the literature as depressive-like behavior. Affective alterations induced by alcohol were generally detected once alcohol exposure ceased, regardless of the animal model used, with few exceptions. It is interesting to note that studies evaluating both acute and chronic abstinence found occurrence of depressive-like behavior in both experimental periods although mostly after prolonged abstinence, which may indicate that the negative affective state as a consequence of abstinence, especially when maintained for prolonged periods, might be a risk factor for displaying depressive-like behavior, analogous to the way in which depression manifests itself in abstinent AUD patients.

2.3 Depression contributes to the risk of alcohol relapse

As previously mentioned, a negative affective state is not only a consequence of consumption but also could represent a maintenance factor for the addiction cycle [28]. In coherence, the "self-medication" theory postulates that the desire to avoid or alleviate preexisting or abstinence-related aversive states is a determining factor of excessive drug use and relapse [48]. Relapse is one of the most complicated components of drug addiction and involves a complex interaction of drug-associated cues that respond to multiple biological, psychiatric, psychological, and psychosocial factors which may precipitate the restoration of consumption [49, 50]. Therefore, one of the main goals in treating substance abuse is to preserve abstinence.

2.4 Clinical evidence of depressive symptomatology contributing to the risk of alcohol relapse

Clinical data strongly support the relevance of negative emotionality in protracted abstinence and relapse. Thus, for example, a higher prevalence of depressed mood has been observed in AUD patients who relapsed [51]. Depression-related low motivation has been shown to precipitate alcohol relapse, while improvements contributed to greater abstinence [52–55]. In fact, those studies have emphasized the need to treat depression to preserve abstinence and improve outcome of patients with AUD. We mentioned before that the AUD can contribute to an ID or a SID. Thus, some authors wonder whether transient symptomatology (SID) would affect consumption in the same way as the observed ID in prolonged abstinence. In this sense, it has been suggested that while affective dysregulation in protracted abstinence is likely to be of immediate relevance for relapse to excessive alcohol use, the link between the early withdrawal phenomena and subsequent affective alterations remains unclear. However, other authors have concluded that both categories should be taken into account as factors that would precipitate relapse. Specifically, SID has been associated with a shorter time for the first alcohol consumption after discharge, while ID, in addition, predicted relapse to alcohol dependence. Interestingly, ID prior to the AUD did not predict outcomes for patients [56].

2.5 Preclinical evidence of depressive-like behavior contributing to the risk of alcohol relapse

Results from clinical studies underline the need to understand possible underlying factors that contribute to the mutual negative influence of both pathologies. In this sense, animal models of AUD and depression offer the possibility of elucidating potential factors involved in the development of dual disorders [57]. Despite the prevalent comorbidity between depression and AUDs, direct evidence of causality of co-occurrence of the two pathologies is still scarce. Thus, Riga et al. [58] used a combination of models of depression and AUD through social defeat and alcohol self-administration and reported that a persistent depressive-like state led to profound alcohol reward-related changes, exaggerating the incentive salience of alcohol and facilitating cue-induced relapse to alcohol seeking. In addition, Lee et al. [47] reported higher alcohol self-administration behavior in mice which exhibited depressive-like behavior in prolonged abstinence as consequence of alcohol self-administration. It is interesting to note that this condition only occurred in animals that were exposed to alcohol during their adolescence and not in those in which the first exposure took place during adulthood, and that did not show alcohol-related affective alterations. Animal studies would show that affective alterations that persist in prolonged abstinence, regardless of whether they were related or not with alcohol exposure, would increase self-administration behavior under alcohol re-exposition.

3. Alcohol use disorders and hippocampal neurogenesis deterioration

Years ago, the proposal arose that alcohol abuse might exert its negative effect in the human brain through an induction of neuronal loss on the hippocampus. In agreement, animal models of chronic alcohol exposure have shown consistently that alcohol is toxic to hippocampal neurons, inducing cell loss. Subsequent studies have led to suggest that alcohol may result in hippocampal pathology and deterioration through effects on adult HN (see [6]).

3.1 Clinical evidence of AUDs contributing to hippocampal neurogenesis deterioration

The lack of techniques to assess adult HN in vivo in AUD patients limits the available information in this regard essentially to postmortem or neuroimaging studies. To date, we have only found one study that has shown that alcohol would have a negative effect on HN in humans [59]. Authors reported reduced numbers of three biomarkers representing different stages of the HN process: Ki67, as marker for cell proliferation, the sex determining region Y-box (Sox2) as stem/progenitor cell marker, and doublecortin (DCX) as marker of neural maturation in the dentate gyrus in subjects with ongoing alcohol abuse. These results converge with previous findings in human with a history of drug abuse [60]. Otherwise, neuroimaging studies allow the detection that alcohol abuse could also impair hippocampal volume. Indeed, some studies have revealed decreases in hippocampal volume in AUD patients, although these changes have been shown to revert with abstinence (reviewed in [61]). There is also evidence of impairment in hippocampus-related functions as consequence of problematic alcohol consumption, effects that, similarly to those found in volumetric studies, could improve with abstinence [62].

3.2 Preclinical evidence of alcohol contributing to hippocampal neurogenesis deterioration

Animal studies are useful to compensate for the limited clinical evidence in AUD patients. In fact, the most consistent evidence of alcohol-induced hippocampal impairment due to, in part, its action on HN comes from preclinical studies. In addition, the different immunolabeling techniques allow us to differentiate the stages of adult animal HN, as proliferation, maturation, migration, and survival of newly generated cells. Obtaining samples throughout different stages offers detailed information on how these processes are altered along the addictive cycle, which constitutes a great advantage over the limitations of postmortem studies in humans. The majority of in vivo studies have shown that alcohol intoxication leads to an overall decrease in HN through alcohol's effects on cell proliferation and survival [63], while those HN parameters show heterogeneous results when assessed throughout abstinence. Several animal studies have evaluated HN parameters along acute withdrawal and/or protracted abstinence in different AUD models. Studies mainly analyzed parameters of HN at different times throughout abstinence and reported increases, decreases, and mixed results in HN-related parameters [64–79]. Studies were mainly in rodents (except [72], done in nonhuman primates). A large part of the studies used a 4-day binge model or self-administration protocols, whereas few authors used the CIE vapor exposure model. Different immunolabeling techniques have been used to assess HN in animals, mainly the thymidine analogue bromodeoxyuridine (BrdU), which is incorporated into dividing cells and allows monitoring of newly generated neurons in the adult brain. Main relevant aspects of results from those studies are analyzed in detail in the conclusion.

3.3 Hippocampal neurogenesis deterioration contributes to the risk of alcohol relapse

Hippocampus is essential in consolidation of stimuli previously paired with drug intake, and authors have proposed that alcohol produces strong deficits in hippocampus-dependent learning and memory and attenuates hippocampal plasticity during withdrawal, which may motivate attempts to self-medicate resulting in relapse and maintenance of drug use [80]. In this sense, one way by which impaired HN could contribute to addiction would be by disrupting learning and memory and by inducing negative affective states, both factors increasing susceptibility to relapse [81]. On the other hand, research during the last decade has shown that it is possible to disrupt alcohol-induced cues and that this has a lasting impact in reducing the tendency to seek drugs and to relapse [82]. In this regard, authors have suggested that although there are a host of plastic changes that occur with abstinence, one way that the hippocampus may recover in abstinence is through the repopulation of the dentate gyrus by adult HN [6].

3.4 Clinical evidence of hippocampal neurogenesis deterioration contributes to the risk of alcohol relapse

In the same way as in the previous sections, human studies provide indirect indicators of the role of HN, such as the volume and functionality of the hippocampus. In this regard, clinical studies found that deficits in hippocampal volume in AUD patients compared with healthy controls normalize over an abstinence period of 2 weeks [83] and that hippocampal volume did not constitute a predictive factor for relapse risk in abstinent alcoholics [84]. On the other hand, it has been observed that the hippocampal-dependent functions could continue to be altered even in prolonged abstinence [62], which could be a factor that, as other authors propose, would alter cognitive aspects linked to the risk of relapse [80]. Information from clinical studies shows that the course of the AUD would be related to the functionality of the hippocampus and not so much with alterations in its structure. Unfortunately, like the previous section, we are faced with a lack of clinical evidence in this regard, since we do not have information on the role that newly generated neurons in the hippocampus would play on the learning and memory processes involved in prevent relapse.

3.5 Preclinical evidence of hippocampal neurogenesis deterioration contributes to the risk of alcohol relapse

Numerous animal studies have led to suggest that low neurogenic states could regulate the addictive behavior, assuming a factor of addiction or comorbid vulnerability [12]. Specifically, animal models of drug addiction studies have led to propose that adult HN appears to be important for the maintenance of hippocampal neuroplasticity, such that reducing HN during abstinence may increase the vulnerability to relapse, while enhancing HN during abstinence may help reduce the risk of relapse [22]. Among the studies cited that assessed HN parameters, only one study [78] analyzed the levels of alcohol consumption after the period of abstinence. Thus, they reported augmented alcohol self-administration after 4 weeks of abstinence in animals that showed reduced HN at the end of the experiment as consequence of a combination of self-administration and vapor exposures to alcohol (dependent animals) compared to animals that showed no reductions in HN who did not receive exposure to vaporized alcohol (nondependent animals). Some results from [78] suggest that the observed reactive HN effect does not have an implication in recovery. On the contrary, animals that showed this reactive effect and lower levels of survival of newly generated neurons ended up showing higher alcohol consumption during relapse. Main implications of these findings are analyzed in the conclusion.

4. AD treatment in alcohol use disorders, depression, and hippocampal neurogenesis

Several studies have led to the suggestion that reversing depressive symptomatology [54] and HN deterioration [21] could be a therapeutical option in cases of comorbidity between AUDs and depression. Given the potential of ADs to improve affective symptoms and promote HN, it is reasonable to assume that such treatment would benefit AUD patients. The following sections attempt to clarify these aspects.

4.1 Clinical evidence of antidepressant treatment improves depressive symptomatology and hippocampal neurogenesis deterioration

Meta-analysis and reviews that integrate results of clinical studies in which patients with AUD and depression were treated with ADs show drug-dependent and inconclusive results. Some findings showed that SSRIs adequately treat depressive symptomatology in individuals with AUD and depression [85–87], while others showed that SSRIs were not more effective than placebo in treating comorbid patients [88, 89]. In relation, it has also been seen that SSRIs would not show greater effects than TCAs [90]. In fact, results from different studies using TCAs seem to converge in its effectiveness in alleviating depressive symptomatology [88, 91]. This may present differences in the response to a treatment for depression in alcohol-dependent participants depending on the different types of depression, as a stronger effect of ADs was found in ID than in SID patients [32]. The most recent meta-analysis available concerning the efficacy of AD treatment in these patients shows a modest effect in some outcomes of depression [92]. However, most authors point out the need for more studies with similar outcome measures, well-defined sample designs, adequate doses, and duration of treatment so that the integration of studies can reach conclusions with a high quality of evidence [87, 90, 92], and some of them emphasize the need to evaluate possible alternative ADs, as, for example, nonselective or partial agonist-reuptake inhibitors [93, 94]. On the other hand, as seen in the introduction, ADs have shown to potentially increase HN in depressed patients [20, 21]. Unfortunately, no evidence of AD-related HN effect has been described in AUD patients.

4.2 Preclinical evidence of antidepressant treatment improves depressive-like behavior and hippocampal neurogenesis deterioration in alcohol exposure and abstinence

Studies in animals have suggested that the ability of AD treatment to affect HN would be linked to its behavioral therapeutic effects [8]. In fact, authors reported that increasing HN has been demonstrated to be necessary and sufficient to reduce depressive-like behavior in animals [95]. On the contrary, other authors have concluded that, although ADs promote HN, this would not be a critical event for their mood-rectifying actions [96]. In the same direction, authors have proposed that the therapeutic effect of the AD would not be determined exclusively by an increase in the number of newly generated neurons but rather in the way in which those neurons are functionally incorporated into hippocampal preexisting circuits that would be linked to recovery [97]. Few animal studies evaluated the efficacy of an AD treatment (desipramine, imipramine, and amitifadine) in a model of alcohol exposure. Studies from Getachew et al. [36, 43] found that subchronic desipramine and imipramine treatment reversed depression-like behavior and anxiety in rodents under acute withdrawal conditions. Similarly, Warnock et al. [39] reported that two different doses of acute amitifadine reversed the abstinence-induced increased immobility in the FST. Finally, Stevenson et al. [37] reported that subchronic desipramine reverted depression-like behavior and restored HN parameters, both aspects impaired under protracted abstinence conditions in mice. Similarly, other studies have tested the efficacy of AD-like drugs as 7,8-DHF, a trkB agonist [40]; trichostatin A, a histone deacetylase inhibitor [76]; rolipram, a phosphodiesterase-4 inhibitor [45]; or ketamine, a N-methyl-D-aspartate receptor antagonist [42, 46], reporting that those treatments also restored the HN parameters and/or the behavioral alterations impaired by the exposure and abstinence to alcohol. In addition, non-pharmacological conditions, as wheel running or natural extracts, induced similar patterns of recovery in HN parameters [65, 77] and in depressive-like behavior [45, 50] in rodents exposed and abstinent of alcohol. This data, in conjunction with previous studies that used ADs, would suggest that if a treatment had protective effects on the NH function, it could also reflect its therapeutic effect on affective disturbances in alcohol exposed animals. Nevertheless, the causality of this relationship needs to be further elucidated. **Figure 2** illustrates the possible state and role of HN during alcohol withdrawal.

4.3 Clinical evidence of antidepressant treatment improves depressive and alcohol use disorder outcome

Although ADs are not among the first-line treatment options in AUD, they are among the additional alternative treatments available, mainly when comorbid

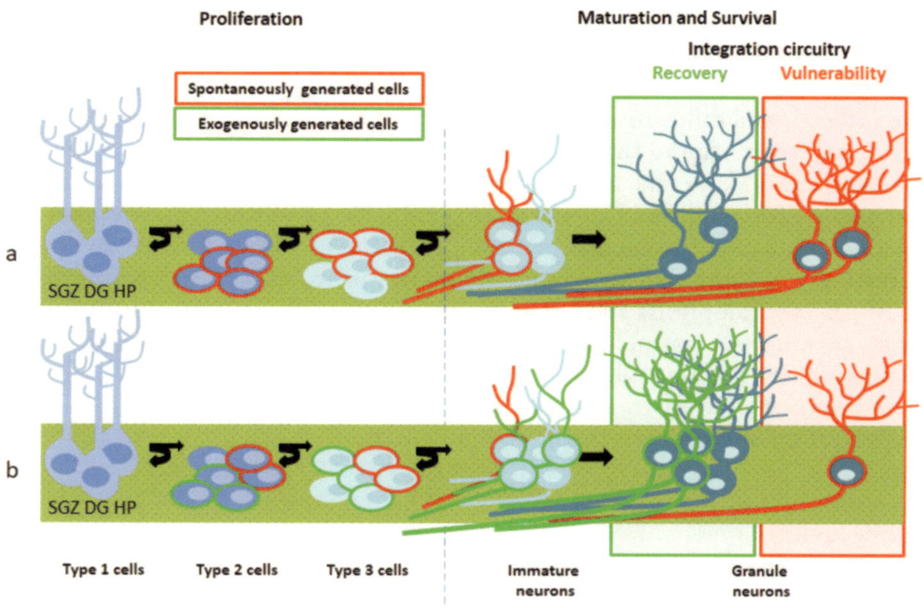

Figure 2.
(a) Schematic representation of the adult HN along alcohol withdrawal and abstinence. Spontaneous burst in cell proliferation is followed by a lower survivability and aberrant patterns of cell migration and integration of the newly generated neurons which could contribute to vulnerability related circuitry. (b) Exogenously induced cell proliferation (by physical exercise or proneurogenic treatment as ADs) could prevent the consolidation of neural circuitry involved in vulnerability, promoting survivability and integration of the newly generated neurons into neural pathways of recovery.

conditions are present [16]. In this regard, authors have proposed that AD treatment could ameliorate alcohol consumption [98], possibly by improving depressive symptoms [99]. Some of the aforementioned studies and meta-analysis evaluated alcohol-related outcomes in AUD depressed patients [87, 90, 92], showing a modest or no efficacy of AD treatment in alleviating some aspects linked to alcohol consumption. Recent conclusions show that ADs increased the number of participants abstaining during the trials and reduced the number of drinks per drinking day, while no differences were reported between ADs and placebo in other relevant outcomes of the AUD [92]. In addition to the mentioned low overall effectiveness, it is important to mention that some studies reported even poorer drinking outcomes in AUD patients treated with SSRIs compared to those treated with placebo [100–102]. In this line, studies have reported clinical cases where treatment with SSRIs appears to be the cause of increased frequency of intoxication by alcohol and new onset of alcohol-related problems [103–105]. Finally, patients who actively drink suffering of comorbid anxiety and AUD have also shown that they may increase alcohol consumption under treatment with SSRIs [106].

4.4 Preclinical evidence of antidepressant treatment improves alcohol relapse

Preclinical data concerning the effectiveness of pharmacological treatments in AUDs is still scarce [107]. Animal studies that evaluate the effect of different AD treatments on preventing alcohol consumption report reduction in alcohol intake after an acute drug dose or under short-term relapse conditions [108]. Nonetheless, taking in mind that the evaluation of the effectiveness of conventional AD treatment should be done considering the delay in its therapeutic effects, studies should go beyond short-term evaluations, assessing long-term consequences of treatment in animal models that better mimic AUD patient conditions [109]. Thus, unlike studies using acute treatments, authors that evaluated chronic and subchronic escitalopram, sertraline, paroxetine, fluoxetine (SSRIs), and duloxetine, dual serotonin/norepinephrine reuptake inhibitor (SNRI) treatments found that, along the treatment period, animals showed lower alcohol intake levels, but cessation of treatment produced a restoration of basal alcohol consumption [110–112]. Ho et al. [110] also found an augmentation in alcohol intake in depressed animals once treatment with escitalopram ceased. Interestingly, authors also found the same effect in animals under combination of AD (escitalopram) and anti-relapse (acamprosate) treatments. Related to that, subchronic treatment with different ADs (SSRIs and SNRIs) has been demonstrated to augment alcohol consumption in animal models of alcohol deprivation, which were treated along abstinence and re-exposed to alcohol self-administration once AD treatment ended [113, 114].

5. Conclusions

Translating evidence from preclinical studies to clinical practice still creates a major challenge in development of new pharmacological treatments in AUDs. The first thing we must point out is the lack of animal studies that have evaluated the effectiveness of the AD treatment in alcohol exposure and abstinence. In this sense, it is important to highlight the numerous studies in animals that evaluate the alcohol exposure and abstinence impact on affective and HN parameters compared to the scarce studies that try to reverse such effects by testing appropriate ADs. In addition, strong criteria are needed when evaluating treatments in AUD animal models, highlighting the use of self-administration procedures and the evaluation of dependence by observing abstinence and relapse behavior. In this sense, animal studies evaluating HN alterations were mainly used as short periods (4 days) of forced alcohol exposition, while prolonged self-administration or CIE models, which better represent important aspects of alcohol consumption patterns in AUD patients, were used to a lesser extent.

One of the most direct methodological limitations when comparing clinical and preclinical studies is determined by the period in which the AD treatment begins. Preclinical studies would indicate that animals can display different affective responses to ADs according to the moment it is administered. In addition, AD cessation could have negative repercussions in alcohol consumption and relapse. While these effects should be further clarified in future studies, clinical trials should take these relevant aspects into account.

The debate about the implication of the new neurons generated in the hippocampus as a consequence of alcohol abstinence continues to be an object of interest. Despite alcohol-induced HN impairments that mainly persist along abstinence, some studies have shown increases in parameters of neural proliferation in animals mainly along early withdrawal periods. First, the possible role of this HN re-establishment effect as factor of recovery was considered, but later studies would even point to opposing hypotheses. In this regard, other findings led to the question whether neurons born during this reactive neurogenic process survive or properly integrate into the existing hippocampal circuitry to provide beneficial effects on hippocampal function and recovery. An early increase in neuronal proliferation induced by abstinence, followed by a reduction in survival in prolonged abstinence, appears to result in an increase in alcohol self-administration. Thus, this apparent AD-induced dual role of HN and the consequent changes in addictive behavior should be elucidated.

To resume, preclinical evidence strongly supports that alcohol consumption and abstinence lead to negative affective states and alterations in HN, some of which may persist in prolonged abstinence. Although affective alterations related to alcohol have been evaluated, there is limited data available concerning the alcohol-induced HN deterioration in clinical patients. Both alcohol-induced depression and changes in HN could be relevant to promote relapse, exacerbating the addictive cycle, although additional studies should clarify this complex interaction. Conventional ADs have been proposed to alleviate affective alterations possibly by promoting HN; thus AUD depressed patients could benefit from its effects. Unfortunately, clinical trials still face several limitations in order to draw reliable conclusions in this regard. Moreover, preclinical studies should bear in mind important methodological aspects onward when translating information regarding the efficacy of AD treatment into AUD patients.

Acknowledgements

The authors are grateful to funding support from Plan Nacional Sobre Drogas (PNSD), ref: 2015/005 to L.O. (Ministerio de Sanidad, Política Social e Igualdad).

Conflict of interest

The authors declare no conflict of interest.

Author details

Antonio Ballesta, Francisco Alén, Fernando Rodríguez de Fonseca,
Raquel Gómez de Heras and Laura Orio*
Department of Psychobiology and Methods in Behavioral Sciences, Faculty of Psychology, Complutense University of Madrid, Madrid, Spain

*Address all correspondence to: lorio@psi.ucm.es

References

[1] American Psychiatric Association. Diagnostic and Statistical Manual of Mental Disorders. Vol. 5. Washington, DC: American Psychiatric Association; 2013

[2] Sullivan LE, Fiellin DA, O'Connor PG. The prevalence and impact of alcohol problems in major depression: A systematic review. The American Journal of Medicine. 2005;**118**(4):330-341. DOI: 10.1016/j.amjmed.2005.01.007

[3] Balu DT, Lucki I. Adult hippocampal neurogenesis: Regulation, functional implications, and contribution to disease pathology. Neuroscience and Biobehavioral Reviews. 2008;**33**(3):232-252. DOI: 10.1016/j.neubiorev.2008.08.007

[4] Baptista P, Andrade JP. Adult hippocampal neurogenesis: Regulation and possible functional and clinical correlates. Frontiers in Neuroanatomy. 2018;**12**:44. DOI: 10.3389/fnana.2018.00044

[5] Sahay A, Hen R. Adult hippocampal neurogenesis in depression. Nat Neurosci. 2007 Sep;**10**(9):1110-1115. DOI: 10.1038/nn1969

[6] Olsufka RA, Peng H, Newton JS, Nixon K. Alcohol effects on adult neural stem cells–A novel mechanism of neurotoxicity and recovery in alcohol use disorders. In: Rasmussen TP, editor. Stem Cells in Birth Defects Research and Developmental Toxicology. Hoboken, NJ: Wiley; 2018. DOI: 10.1002/9781119283249.ch8

[7] Jacobs BL, van Praag H, Gage FH. Adult brain neurogenesis and psychiatry: A novel theory of depression. Molecular Psychiatry. 2000;**5**:262-269

[8] Tanti A, Belzung C. Hippocampal neurogenesis: A biomarker for depression or antidepressant effects? Methodological considerations and perspectives for future research. Cell and Tissue Research. 2013;**354**(1):203-219. DOI: 10.1007/s00441-013-1612-z

[9] Peng L, Bonaguidi MA. Function and dysfunction of adult hippocampal neurogenesis in regeneration and disease. The American Journal of Pathology. 2018 Jan;**188**(1):23-28. DOI: 10.1016/j.ajpath.2017.09.004

[10] Renoir T, Pang TY, Lanfumey L. Drug withdrawal-induced depression: Serotonergic and plasticity changes in animal models. Neuroscience & Biobehavioral Reviews. 2012;**36**(1):696-726. DOI: 10.1016/j.neubiorev.2011.10.003

[11] Crews FT, Nixon K. Mechanisms of neurodegeneration and regeneration in alcoholism. Alcohol and Alcoholism. 2009;**44**(2):115-127. DOI: 10.1093/alcalc/agn079

[12] Chambers RA. Adult hippocampal neurogenesis in the pathogenesis of addiction and dual diagnosis disorders. Drug and Alcohol Dependence. 2013;**130**(1-3):1-12. DOI: 10.1016/j.drugalcdep.2012.12.005

[13] Mandyam CD, Koob GF. The addicted brain craves new neurons: Putative role for adult-born progenitors in promoting recovery. Trends in Neurosciences. 2012;**35**(4):250-260. DOI: 10.1016/j.tins.2011.12.005

[14] Abbing-Karahagopian V, Huerta C, Souverein PC, de Abajo F, Leufkens HGM, Slattery J, et al. Antidepressant prescribing in five European countries: Application of common definitions to assess the prevalence, clinical observations, and methodological implications. European Journal of Clinical Pharmacology. 2014;**70**(7):849-857. DOI: 10.1007/s00228-014-1676-z

[15] Marcinkiewcz CA, Lowery-Gionta EG, Kash TL. Serotonin's complex role in alcoholism: Implications for treatment and future research. Alcoholism, Clinical and Experimental Research. 2016 Jun;**40**(6):1192-1201. DOI: 10.1111/acer.13076

[16] Soyka M, Müller CA. Pharmacotherapy of alcoholism—An update on approved and off-label medications. Expert Opinion on Pharmacotherapy. 2017;**18**(12):1187-1199. DOI: 10.1080/14656566.2017.1349098

[17] Schildkraut JJ. The catecholamine hypothesis of affective disorders: A review of supporting evidence. The Journal of Neuropsychiatry and Clinical Neurosciences. 1995 Fall;7(4):524-533; discussion 523-4

[18] Duman RS, Nakagawa S, Malberg J. Regulation of adult neurogenesis by antidepressant treatment. Neuropsychopharmacology. 2001;**25**(6):836-844

[19] Mahar I, Bambico FR, Mechawar N, Nobrega JN. Stress, serotonin, and hippocampal neurogenesis in relation to depression and antidepressant effects. Neuroscience and Biobehavioral Reviews. 2014;**38**:173-192. DOI: 10.1016/j.neubiorev.2013.11.009

[20] Boldrini M, Underwood MD, Hen R, Rosoklija GB, Dwork AJ, Mann JJ, et al. Antidepressants increase neural progenitor cells in the human hippocampus. Neuropsychopharmacology. 2009;**34**(11):2376-2389. DOI: 10.1038/npp.2009.75

[21] Boldrini M, Hen R, Underwood MD, Rosoklija GB, Dwork AJ, Mann JJ, et al. Hippocampal angiogenesis and progenitor cell proliferation are increased with antidepressant use in major depression. Biological Psychiatry. 2012;**72**(7):562-571. DOI: 10.1016/j.biopsych.2012.04.024

[22] Boldrini M, Butt TH, Santiago AN, Tamir H, Dwork AJ, Rosoklija GB, et al. Benzodiazepines and the potential trophic effect of antidepressants on dentate gyrus cells in mood disorders. The International Journal of Neuropsychopharmacology. 2014;**17**(12):1923-1933. DOI: 10.1017/s1461145714000844

[23] Boldrini M, Santiago AN, Hen R, Dwork AJ, Rosoklija GB, Tamir H, et al. Hippocampal granule neuron number and dentate gyrus volume in antidepressant-treated and untreated major depression. Neuropsychopharmacology. 2013 May;**38**(6):1068-1077. DOI: 10.1038/npp.2013.5

[24] Malberg JE, Eisch AJ, Nestler EJ, Duman RS. Chronic antidepressant treatment increases neurogenesis in adult rat hippocampus. The Journal of Neuroscience. 2000;**20**(24):9104-9110

[25] Kempermann G, Gage FH, Aigner L, Song H, Curtis MA, Thuret S, et al. Human adult neurogenesis: Evidence and remaining questions. Cell Stem Cell. 2018;**23**(1):25-30. DOI: 10.1016/j.stem.2018.04.004

[26] Eliwa H, Belzung C, Surget A. Adult hippocampal neurogenesis: Is it the alpha and omega of antidepressant action? Biochemical Pharmacology. 2017;**141**:86-99. DOI: 10.1016/j.bcp.2017.08.005

[27] Hershon HI. Alcohol withdrawal symptoms and drinking behavior. Journal of Studies on Alcohol. 1977;**38**(5):953-971

[28] Koob GF. The dark side of emotion: The addiction perspective. European Journal of Pharmacology. 2015;**753**:73-87. DOI: 10.1016/j.ejphar.2014.11.044

[29] Conner KR, Pinquart M, Gamble SA. Meta-analysis of depression and substance use among individuals with alcohol use disorders. Journal of Substance Abuse Treatment. 2009;**37**(2):127-137. DOI: 10.1016/j.jsat.2008.11.007

[30] Brennan PL, SooHoo S, Lemke S, Schutte KK. Alcohol use predicts 10-year depressive symptom trajectories in the health and retirement study. Journal of Aging and Health. 2016;**28**(5):911-932. DOI: 10.1177/0898264315615837

[31] Skogen JC, Knudsen AK, Hysing M, Wold B, Sivertsen B. Trajectories of alcohol use and association with symptoms of depression from early to late adolescence: The Norwegian Longitudinal Health Behaviour Study. Drug and Alcohol Review. 2016;**35**(3):307-316. DOI: 10.1111/dar.12350

[32] Foulds JA, Adamson SJ, Boden JM, Williman JA, Mulder RT. Depression in patients with alcohol use disorders: Systematic review and meta-analysis of outcomes for independent and substance-induced disorders. Journal of Affective Disorders. 2015;**185**:47-59. DOI: 10.1016/j.jad.2015.06.024

[33] Brown RA, Ramsey SE, Kahler CW, Palm KM, Monti PM, Abrams D, et al. A randomized controlled trial of cognitive-behavioral treatment for depression versus relaxation training for alcohol-dependent individuals with elevated depressive symptoms. Journal of Studies on Alcohol and Drugs. 2011;**72**:286. DOI: 10.15288/jsad.2011.72.286

[34] Foulds JA, Douglas Sellman J, Adamson SJ, Boden JM, Mulder RT, Joyce PR. Depression outcome in alcohol dependent patients: An evaluation of the role of independentand substance-induced depression and other predictors. Journal of Affective Disorders. 2015;**174**:503-510. DOI: 10.1016/j.jad.2014.11.052

[35] Bahorik AL, Leibowitz A, Sterling SA, Travis A, Weisner C, Satre DD. The role of hazardous drinking reductions in predicting depression and anxiety symptom improvement among psychiatry patients: A longitudinal study. Journal of Affective Disorders. 2016;**206**:169-173. DOI: 10.1016/j.jad.2016.07.039

[36] Getachew B, Hauser SR, Taylor RE, Tizabi Y. Desipramine blocks alcohol-induced anxiety- and depressive-like behaviors in two rat strains. Pharmacology, Biochemistry, and Behavior. 2008;**91**:97-103. DOI: 10.1016/j.pbb.2008.06.016

[37] Stevenson JR, Schroeder JP, Nixon K, Besheer J, Crews FT, Hodge CW. Abstinence following alcohol drinking produces depression-like behavior and reduced hippocampal neurogenesis in mice. Neuropsychopharmacology. 2009;**34**:1209-1222. DOI: 10.1038/npp.2008.90

[38] Ehlers CL, Liu W, Wills DN, Crews FT. Periadolescent ethanol vapor exposure persistently reduces measures of hippocampal neurogenesis that are associated with behavioral outcomes in adulthood. Neuroscience. 2013;**244**:1-15. DOI: 10.1016/j.neuroscience.2013.03.058

[39] Warnock KT, Yang ARST, Yi HS, June HL, Kelly T, Basile AS, et al. Amitifadine, a triple monoamine uptake inhibitor, reduces binge drinking and negative affect in an animal model of co-occurring alcoholism and depression symptomatology. Pharmacology Biochemistry and Behavior. 2012;**103**(1):111-118. DOI: 10.1016/j.pbb.2012.07.014

[40] Briones TL, Woods J. Chronic binge-like alcohol consumption in adolescence causes depression-like symptoms

possibly mediated by the effects of BDNF on neurogenesis. Neuroscience. 2013;**254**:324-334. DOI: 10.1016/j.neuroscience.2013.09.031

[41] Pang TY, Renoir T, Du X, Lawrence AJ, Hannan AJ. Depression-related behaviours displayed by female C57BL/6J mice during abstinence from chronic ethanol consumption are rescued by wheel-running. The European Journal of Neuroscience. 2013;**37**(11):1803-1810. DOI: 10.1111/ejn.12195

[42] Holleran KM, Wilson HH, Fetterly TL, et al. Ketamine and MAG lipase inhibitor-dependent reversal of evolving depressive-like behavior during forced abstinence from alcohol drinking. Neuropsychopharmacology. 2016;**41**(8):2062-2071. DOI: 10.1038/npp.2016.3

[43] Getachew B, Hauser SR, Csoka AB11, Taylor RE, Tizabi Y. Role of cortical alpha-2 adrenoceptors in alcohol withdrawal-induced depression and tricyclic antidepressants. Drug and Alcohol Dependence. 2017;**175**:133-139. DOI: 10.1016/j.drugalcdep.2017.03.004

[44] Kim HJ, Park SD, Lee RM, Lee BH, Choi SH, Hwang SH, et al. Gintonin attenuates depressive-like behaviors associated with alcohol withdrawal in mice. Journal of Affective Disorders. 2017;**215**:23-29. DOI: 10.1016/j.jad.2017.03.026

[45] Gong MF, Wen RT, Xu Y, Pan JC, Fei N, Zhou YM, et al. Attenuation of ethanol abstinence-induced anxiety- and depressive-like behavior by the phosphodiesterase-4 inhibitor rolipram in rodents. Psychopharmacology. 2017;**234**(20):3143-3151. DOI: 10.1007/s00213-017-4697-3

[46] Vranjkovic O, Winkler G, Winder DG. Ketamine administration during a critical period after forced ethanol abstinence inhibits the development of time-dependent affective disturbances. Neuropsychopharmacology. 2018 Aug;**43**(9):1915-1923. DOI: 10.1038/s41386-018-0102-0

[47] Lee KM, Coehlo MA, Solton NR, Szumlinski KK. Negative affect and excessive alcohol intake incubate during protracted withdrawal from binge-drinking in adolescent, but not adult mice. Frontiers in Psychology. 2017;**8**:1128. DOI: 10.3389/fpsyg.2017.01128

[48] Markou A, Kosten TR, Koob GF. Neurobiological similarities in depression and drug dependence: A self-medication hypothesis. Neuropsychopharmacology. 1998;**18**(3):135-174

[49] Durazzo TC, Meyerhoff DJ. Psychiatric, demographic, and brain morphological predictors of relapse after treatment for an alcohol use disorder. Alcoholism, Clinical and Experimental Research. 2016;**41**(1):107. DOI: 116. 10.1111/acer.13267

[50] Milton AL, Everitt BJ. The psychological and neurochemical mechanisms of drug memory reconsolidation: Implications for the treatment of addiction. The European Journal of Neuroscience. 2010;**31**(12):2308-2319. DOI: 10.1111/j.1460-9568.2010.07249.x

[51] Strowig AB. Relapse determinants reported by men treated for alcohol addiction: The prominence of depressed mood. Journal of Substance Abuse Treatment. 2000 Dec;**19**(4):469-474

[52] Cengisiz C, Deveci A, Yapici A. Effects of depression on treatment motivation in male alcohol dependence. Noro Psikiyatri Arsivi. 2015;**52**(4):412-416. DOI: 10.5152/npa.2015.9859

[53] Holzhauer CG, Gamble SA. Depressive symptoms mediate the relationship between changes in

emotion regulation during treatment and abstinence among women with alcohol use disorders. Psychology of Addictive Behaviors. 2017;**31**(3): 284-294. DOI: 10.1037/adb0000274

[54] Suter M, Strik W, Moggi F. Depressive symptoms as a predictor of alcohol relapse after residential treatment programs for alcohol use disorder. Journal of Substance Abuse Treatment. 2011;**41**(3):225-232. DOI: 10.1016/j.jsat.2011.03.005

[55] Heilig M, Egli M, Crabbe JC, Becker HC. Acute withdrawal, protracted abstinence and negative affect in alcoholism: Are they linked? Addiction Biology. 2010;**15**(2):169-184. DOI: 10.1111/j.1369-1600.2009.00194.x

[56] Samet S, Fenton MC, Nunes E, Greenstein E, Aharonovich E, Hasin D. Effects of independent and substance-induced major depressive disorder on remission and relapse of alcohol, cocaine and heroin dependence. Addiction. 2012;**108**(1):115-123. DOI: 10.1111/j.1360-0443.2012.04010.x

[57] Ng E, Browne CJ, Samsom JN, AHC W. Depression and substance use comorbidity: What we have learned from animal studies. The American Journal of Drug and Alcohol Abuse. 2017;**43**(4):456-474. DOI: 10.1080/00952990.2016.1183020

[58] Riga D, Schmitz LJ, van der Harst JE, van Mourik Y, Hoogendijk WJ, Smit AB, et al. A sustained depressive state promotes a guanfacine reversible susceptibility to alcohol seeking in rats. Neuropsychopharmacology. 2014;**39**(5):1115-1124. DOI: 10.1038/npp.2013.311

[59] Le Maître TW, Dhanabalan G, Bogdanovic N, Alkass K, Druid H. Effects of alcohol abuse on proliferating cells, stem/progenitor cells, and immature neurons in the adult human hippocampus. Neuropsychopharmacology. 2018;**43**(4):690-699. DOI: 10.1038/npp.2017.251

[60] Bayer R, Franke H, Ficker C, Richter M, Lessig R, Büttner A, et al. Alterations of neuronal precursor cells in stages of human adult neurogenesis in heroin addicts. Drug and Alcohol Dependence. 2015;**156**:139-149. DOI: 10.1016/j.drugalcdep.2015.09.005

[61] Wilson S, Bair JL, Thomas KM, Iacono WG. Problematic alcohol use and reduced hippocampal volume: A meta-analytic review. Psychological Medicine. 2017;**47**(13):2288-2301. DOI: 10.1017/S0033291717000721

[62] Staples MC, Mandyam CD. Thinking after drinking: Impaired hippocampal-dependent cognition in human alcoholics and animal models of alcohol dependence. Frontiers in Psychiatry. 2016;**7**:162. DOI: 10.3389/fpsyt.2016.00162

[63] Xu C, Loh HH, Law PY. Effects of addictive drugs on adult neural stem/progenitor cells. Cellular and Molecular Life Sciences. 2015;**73**(2):327-348. DOI: 10.1007/s00018-015-2067-z

[64] Nixon K, Kim DH, Potts EN, He J, Crews FT. Distinct cell proliferation events during abstinence after alcohol dependence: Microglia proliferation precedes neurogenesis. Neurobiology of Disease. 2008;**31**(2):218-229. DOI: 10.1016/j.nbd.2008.04.009

[65] Maynard ME, Leasure JL. Exercise enhances hippocampal recovery following binge ethanol exposure. PLoS ONE. 2013;**8**(9):e76644. DOI: 10.1371/journal.pone.0076644

[66] McClain JA, Morris SA, Marshall SA, Nixon K. Ectopic hippocampal neurogenesis in adolescent male rats following alcohol dependence.

Addiction Biology. 2013;**19**(4):687-699. DOI: 10.1111/adb.12075

[67] Nickell CRG, Peng H, Hayes DM, Chen KY, McClain JA, Nixon K. Type 2 neural progenitor cell activation drives reactive neurogenesis after binge-like alcohol exposure in adolescent male rats. Frontiers in Psychiatry. 2017;**8**:283. DOI: 10.3389/fpsyt.2017.00283

[68] Hayes DM, Nickell CG, Chen KY, McClain JA, Heath MM, Deeny MA, et al. Activation of neural stem cells from quiescence drives reactive hippocampal neurogenesis after alcohol dependence. Neuropharmacology. 2018;**133**:276-288. DOI: 10.1016/j.neuropharm.2018.01.032

[69] Hansson AC, Nixon K, Rimondini R, et al. Long-term suppression of forebrain neurogenesis and loss of neuronal progenitor cells following prolonged alcohol dependence in rats. The International Journal of Neuropsychopharmacology. 2010;**13**(5):583-593. DOI: 10.1017/S1461145710000246

[70] Crews FT, Mdzinarishvili A, Kim D, He J, Nixon K. Neurogenesis in adolescent brain is potently inhibited by ethanol. Neuroscience. 2006;**137**(2):437-445. DOI: 10.1016/j.neuroscience.2005.08.090

[71] Richardson HN, Chan SH, Crawford EF, Lee YK, Funk CK, Koob GF, et al. Permanent impairment of birth and survival of cortical and hippocampal proliferating cells following excessive drinking during alcohol dependence. Neurobiology of Disease. 2009;**36**(1): 1-10. DOI: 10.1016/j.nbd.2009.05.021

[72] Taffe MA, Kotzebue RW, Crean RD, Crawford EF, Edwards S, Mandyam CD. Long-lasting reduction in hippocampal neurogenesis by alcohol consumption in adolescent nonhuman primates. Proceedings of the National Academy of Sciences. 2010;**107**(24):11104-11109. DOI: 10.1073/pnas.0912810107

[73] Broadwater MA, Liu W, Crews FT, Spear LP. Persistent loss of hippocampal neurogenesis and increased cell death following adolescent, but not adult chronic ethanol exposure. Developmental Neuroscience. 2014;**36**(3-4):297-305. DOI: 10.1159/000362874

[74] Vetreno RP, Crews FT. Binge ethanol exposure during adolescence leads to a persistent loss of neurogenesis in the dorsal and ventral hippocampus that is associated with impaired adult cognitive functioning. Frontiers in Neuroscience. 2015;**9**:35. DOI: 10.3389/fnins.2015.00035

[75] Morris SA, Eaves DW, Smith AR, Nixon K. Alcohol inhibition of neurogenesis: A mechanism of hippocampal neurodegeneration in an adolescent alcohol abuse model. Hippocampus. 2010;**20**(5):596-607. DOI: 10.1002/hipo.20665

[76] Sakharkar AJ, Vetreno RP, Zhang H, Kokare DM, Crews FT, Pandey SC. A role for histone acetylation mechanisms in adolescent alcohol exposure-induced deficits in hippocampal brain-derived neurotrophic factor expression and neurogenesis markers in adulthood. Brain Structure and Function. 2016;**221**(9):4691-4703. DOI: 10.1007/s00429-016-1196-y

[77] Vetreno RP, Lawrimore CJ, Rowsey PJ, Crews FT. Persistent adult neuroimmune activation and loss of hippocampal neurogenesis following adolescent ethanol exposure: Blockade by exercise and the anti-inflammatory drug indomethacin. Frontiers in Neuroscience. 2018;**12**. DOI: 10.3389/fnins.2018.00200

[78] Somkuwar SS, Fannon MJ, Staples MC, Zamora-Martinez ER, Navarro AI, Kim A, et al. Alcohol

dependence-induced regulation of the proliferation and survival of adult brain progenitors is associated with altered BDNF-TrkB signaling. Brain Structure & Function. 2016;**221**(9):4319-4335. DOI: 10.1007/s00429-015-1163-z

[79] Liu W, Crews FT. Persistent decreases in adult subventricular and hippocampal neurogenesis following adolescent intermittent ethanol exposure. Frontiers in Behavioral Neuroscience. 2017;**11**:151. DOI: 10.3389/fnbeh.2017.00151

[80] Kutlu MG, Gould TJ. Effects of drugs of abuse on hippocampal plasticity and hippocampus-dependent learning and memory: Contributions to development and maintenance of addiction. Learning & Memory. 2016;**23**(10):515-533. DOI: 10.1101/lm.042192.116

[81] Canales JJ. Deficient plasticity in the hippocampus and the spiral of addiction: Focus on adult neurogenesis. Current Topics in Behavioral Neurosciences. 2013;**15**:293-312. DOI: 10.1007/7854_2012_230

[82] Cui C, Noronha A, Warren K, Koob GF, Sinha R, Thakkar M, et al. Brain pathways to recovery from alcohol dependence. Alcohol (Fayetteville, N.Y.). 2015;**49**(5):435-452. DOI: 10.1016/j.alcohol.2015.04.006

[83] Kühn S, Charlet K, Schubert F, Kiefer F, Zimmermann P, Heinz A, et al. Plasticity of hippocampal subfield volume cornu ammonis 2+3 over the course of withdrawal in patients with alcohol dependence. JAMA Psychiatry. 2014;**71**(7):806-811. DOI: 10.1001/jamapsychiatry.2014.352

[84] Gross CM, Spiegelhalder K, Mercak J, Feige B, Langosch JM. Predictability of alcohol relapse by hippocampal volumetry and psychometric variables. Psychiatry Research. 2013;**212**(1):14-18. DOI: 10.1016/j.pscychresns.2012.09.011

[85] Danovitch I, Steiner AJ, Kazdan A, Goldenberg M, Haglund M, Mirocha J, et al. Analysis of patient-reported outcomes of quality of life and functioning before and after treatment of major depressive disorder comorbid with alcohol use disorders. Journal of Addiction Medicine. 2017;**11**(1):47-54. DOI: 10.1097/adm.0000000000000268

[86] Davis LL, Wisniewski SR, Howland RH, Trivedi MH, Husain MM, Fava M, et al. Does comorbid substance use disorder impair recovery from major depression with SSRI treatment? An analysis of the STAR*D level one treatment outcomes. Drug and Alcohol Dependence. 2010;**107**(2-3):161-170. DOI: 10.1016/j.drugalcdep.2009.10.003

[87] Nunes EV, Levin FR. Treatment of depression in patients with alcohol or other drug dependence: A meta-analysis. JAMA. 2004;**291**(15):1887-1896. DOI: 10.1001/jama.291.15.1887

[88] Iovieno N, Tedeschini E, Bentley KH, Evins AE, Papakostas GI. Antidepressants for major depressive disorder and dysthymic disorder in patients with comorbid alcohol use disorders: A meta-analysis of placebo-controlled randomized trials. The Journal of Clinical Psychiatry. 2011;**72**(8):1144-1151. DOI: 10.4088/JCP.10m06217

[89] Zhou X, Qin B, Del Giovane C, Pan J, Gentile S, Liu Y, et al. Efficacy and tolerability of antidepressants in the treatment of adolescents and young adults with depression and substance use disorders: A systematic review and meta-analysis. Addiction. 2015;**110**(1):38-48. DOI: 10.1111/add.12698.10

[90] Torrens M, Fonseca F, Mateu G, Farré M. Efficacy of antidepressants in substance use disorders with and without comorbid depression. A systematic review and meta-analysis. Drug and Alcohol Dependence.

2005;**78**(1):1-22. DOI: 10.1016/j.drugalcdep.2004.09.004

[91] Cornelius J, Chung T, Douaihy A, Kirisci L, Glance J, Kmiec J, et al. A review of the literature of mirtazapine in co-occurring depression and an alcohol use disorder. Journal of Addictive Behaviors, Therapy & Rehabilitation. 2016;**5**(4):159. DOI: 10.4172/2324-9005.1000159

[92] Agabio R, Trogu E, Pani PP. Antidepressants for the treatment of people with co-occurring depression and alcohol dependence. Cochrane Database of Systematic Reviews. 2018;**4**. Art. No.: CD008581. DOI: 10.1002/14651858.CD008581.pub2

[93] Nunes EV, Levin FR. Treatment of co-occurring depression and substance dependence: Using meta-analysis to guide clinical recommendations. Psychiatric Annals. 2008;**38**(11)

[94] Belmer A, Patkar OL, Pitman KM, Bartlett SE. Serotonergic neuroplasticity in alcohol addiction. Brain Plasticity. 2016;**1**(2):177-206. DOI: 10.3233/BPL-150022

[95] Hill AS, Sahay A, Hen R. Increasing adult hippocampal neurogenesis is sufficient to reduce anxiety and depression-like behaviors. Neuropsychopharmacology. 2015;**40**(10):2368-2378. DOI: 10.1038/npp.2015.85

[96] Bessa JM, Ferreira D, Melo I, Marques F, Cerqueira JJ, Palha JA, et al. The mood-improving actions of antidepressants do not depend on neurogenesis but are associated with neuronal remodeling. Molecular Psychiatry. 2009;**14**(8):764-773. DOI: 10.1038/mp.2008.119

[97] Mateus-Pinheiro A, Pinto L, Bessa JM, Morais M, Alves ND, Monteiro S, et al. Sustained remission from depressive-like behavior depends on hippocampal neurogenesis. Translational Psychiatry. 2013;**3**(1):e210. DOI: 10.1038/tp.2012.141

[98] Graham K, Massak A. Alcohol consumption and the use of antidepressants. CMAJ. 2007;**176**(5):633-637. DOI: 10.1503/cmaj.060446

[99] Mann K. Pharmacotherapy of alcohol dependence: A review of the clinical data. CNS Drugs. 2004;**18**(8):485-504. DOI: 10.2165/00023210-200418080-00002

[100] Charney DA, Heath LM, Zikos E, Palacios-Boix J, Gill KJ. Poorer drinking outcomes with citalopram treatment for alcohol dependence: A randomized, double-blind, placebo-controlled trial. Alcoholism, Clinical and Experimental Research. 2015;**39**(9):1756-1765. DOI: 10.1111/acer.12802

[101] Chick J, Aschauer H, Hornik K. Efficacy of fluvoxamine in preventing relapse in alcohol dependence: A one-year, double-blind, placebo-controlled multicentre study with analysis by typology. Drug and Alcohol Dependence. 2004;**74**(1):61-70. DOI: 10.1016/j.drugalcdep.2003.11.012

[102] Dundon W, Lynch KG, Pettinati HM, Lipkin C. Treatment outcomes in type A and B alcohol dependence 6 months after serotonergic pharmacotherapy. Alcoholism: Clinical and Experimental Research. 2004;**28**:1065-1073. DOI: 10.1097/01.alc.0000130974.50563.04

[103] Atigari OV, Kelly AM, Jabeen Q, Healy D. New onset alcohol dependence linked to treatment with selective serotonin reuptake inhibitors. The International Journal of Risk & Safety in Medicine. 2013;**25**(105-109). DOI: 10.3233/JRS-130586

[104] Brookwell L, Hogana C, Healya D, Manginb D. Ninety-three cases of alcohol dependence following SSRI treatment. The International Journal of Risk & Safety in Medicine. 2014;**26**: 99-107. DOI: 10.3233/JRS-140616

[105] Menkes DB, Herxheimer A. Interaction between antidepressants and alcohol: Signal amplification by multiple case reports. The International Journal of Risk & Safety in Medicine. 2014;**26**(3):163-170. DOI: 10.3233/JRS-140632

[106] Gimeno C, Dorado ML, Roncero C, Szerman N, Vega P, Balanzá-Martínez V, et al. Treatment of comorbid alcohol dependence and anxiety disorder: Review of the scientific evidence and recommendations for treatment. Frontiers in Psychiatry. 2017;**8**:173. DOI: 10.3389/fpsyt.2017.00173

[107] Barajaz AM, Kliethermes CL. An assessment of the utilization of the preclinical rodent model literature in clinical trials of putative therapeutics for the treatment of alcohol use disorders. Drug and Alcohol Dependence. 2017;**181**:77-84. DOI: 10.1016/j.drugalcdep.2017.09.022

[108] Simon O'Brien E, Legastelois R, Houchi H, Vilpoux C, Alaux-Cantin S, Pierrefiche O, et al. Fluoxetine, desipramine, and the dual antidepressant milnacipran reduce alcohol self-administration and/or relapse in dependent rats. Neuropsychopharmacology. 2011;**36**: 1518-1530. DOI: 10.1038/npp.2011.37

[109] Bell RL, Hauser SR, Liang T, Sari Y, Maldonado-Devincci A, Rodd ZA. Rat animal models for screening medications to treat alcohol use disorders. Neuropharmacology. 2017;**122**:201-243. DOI: 10.1016/j.neuropharm.2017.02.004

[110] Ho AMC, Qiu Y, Jia YF, Aguiar FS, Hinton DJ, Karpyak VM, et al. Combined effects of acamprosate and escitalopram on ethanol consumption in mice. Alcoholism, Clinical and Experimental Research. 2016;**40**(7):1531-1539. DOI: 10.1111/acer.13099

[111] Gulley JM, McNamara C, Barbera TJ, Ritz MC, George FR. Selective serotonin reuptake inhibitors: Effects of chronic treatment on ethanol-reinforced behavior in mice. Alcohol. 1995;**12**(3):177-181. DOI: 10.1016/0741-8329(94)00079-s

[112] Skelly MJ, Weiner JL. Chronic treatment with prazosin or duloxetine lessens concurrent anxiety-like behavior and alcohol intake: Evidence of disrupted noradrenergic signaling in anxiety-related alcohol use. Brain and Behavior. 2014;**4**(4):468-483. DOI: 10.1002/brb3.230

[113] Alén F, Orio L, Gorriti MA, de Heras RG, Ramírez-López MT, Pozo MA, et al. Increased alcohol consumption in rats after subchronic antidepressant treatment. The International Journal of Neuropsychopharmacology. 2013;**16**:1809-1818. DOI: 10.1017/s1461145713000217

[114] Alén F, Serrano A, Gorriti MÁ, Pavón FJ, Orio L, de Heras RG, et al. The administration of atomoxetine during alcohol deprivation induces a time-limited increase in alcohol consumption after relapse. The International Journal of Neuropsychopharmacology. 2014;**17**(11):1905-1910. DOI: 10.1017/s146114571400087x

Chapter 3

Resistant Depression

Jose Alfonso Ontiveros

Abstract

The term resistant points out a clinical phenomenon in which there is a lack of response to one or more therapeutic interventions. Resistance to major depressive disorder treatment causes distress to patients and their relatives, and increases the number of hospital admissions, outpatient consultations, use of psychoactive drugs, and treatment costs. Despite its serious medical and psychosocial medical implications, the definition of treatment resistant depression continues to be ambiguous and controversial. The lack of an agreement on definition, as well as the research on the subject being difficult, limits the practical knowledge on the best treatment options for groups of treatment resistant depression (TRD) patients. We review the concept and definitions of treatment resistant depression as well as the medical literature on different treatment methods studied and comparative studies. Finally, some relevant neurobiological data are reviewed.

Keywords: treatment, major depressive disorder, resistant depression, antidepressants, review

1. Introduction

The term "resistant" is widely employed in medical practice to point out a clinical phenomenon in which there is a lack of response to one or more therapeutic interventions. The presence of treatment resistance implies a specific series of clinical interventions, typically multidisciplinary, and focuses on solving or minimizing a medical problem. Resistance to major depressive disorder treatment, but also to other depressive disorders, such as dysthymia and bipolar depression, causes distress to patients and their relatives, and increases the number of hospital admissions, outpatient consultations, the use of psychoactive drugs, and treatment costs up to six times [1]. The definition of treatment resistant depression (TRD) continues to be ambiguous and controversial despite its serious medical and psychosocial implications. In medical literature, we can find more than 10 different definitions [2]. Many authors have published staging systems with their own definitions, descriptions, and characteristics on TRD [3–7]. The most accepted definition is a lack of response to two different pharmacological classes of antidepressants [8]. However, this definition may seem simplistic today as published treatment results on TRD patients emerge. The lack of an agreed TRD definition as well as the difficulties to do research on the subject limit our practical knowledge on the best treatment options for groups of TRD patients.

We review the concept and definitions of TRD. We also review the medical literature on different treatment methods studied as well as comparative studies. Finally, we review some relevant emerging neurobiological data.

2. Treatment resistance depression (TRD)

2.1 The concept of resistant depression

Although this phenomenon had already been described, many authors have introduced the concept of TRD since 1974 [9, 10]. This concept arises at a time when there were only tricyclic, tetracyclic, and monoamine-oxidase inhibitors (MAOIs) antidepressants available. In spite of its importance, the definition of treatment resistance regarding major depression continues to be a wide and inconsistent notion. A review of the literature identifies a range of definitions for TRD that go from non-response to a single antidepressant (for 4 or more weeks) to lack of response to different classes of antidepressants and electroconvulsive therapy (ECT) [2]. Treatment should be appropriate in dose and duration [2, 11–13], and patients must have full compliance to it [13] to consider a patient as resistant to treatment. There is no consensus on the number of treatments and when these are indicators of resistance.

A dichotomic denomination has been proposed for resistant depression, viz. an absolute and a relative. Absolute resistance is an inappropriate anti-depressive response toward a treatment given for an appropriate period of time at the maximum non-toxic dose. On the other hand, relative resistance to treatment is defined when this is given at a suboptimal dose or duration [5, 10, 14]. The terms "chronic," "refractory," and "difficult-to-treat depression" have been employed as synonyms in the absence of a nonspecific number of clinical trials for one or more antidepressants. Treatment refractory depression refers to major depression that does not respond to multiple sequential treatments. There is no clear difference between treatment resistant depression and refractory depression [5, 8, 11]. Chronicity, however, refers to a pathological clinical phenomenon that lasts for 2 or more years. There is no consensus on depressive symptom severity to consider it as resistant. It has been suggested that a score of 16 or more on the Hamilton depression 17-item scale (HAM-D) is enough to confirm the diagnosis. However, patients with persistent mild or moderate depressive symptoms may have a worse prognosis than those in remission [15]. The definition of Berlim and Turecki [2], which considers TRD as an episode of major depression that has not improved after two proper attempts with different classes of antidepressants, prevails today. The European Medicine Agency (EMA), on a TRD definition review, considers it as a clinically relevant major depression that has not benefited from at least two appropriate attempts of treatment with at least two antidepressants with a different action mechanism [16]. The definition which considers TRD as an episode of major depression that has not improved after two proper attempts with different classes of antidepressants [2] seems to be backed up by the STAR*D study, which shows that improvement chances diminish after the second treatment failure [17, 18]. Treatment resistance to pharmacologic treatment seems to move on a continuum that ranges from total response to total resistance to therapeutic intervention and not as an all-or-nothing phenomenon [5, 19, 20]. However, no definition has been investigated regarding validity and predictability [5, 21]. Inconsistencies on the definition not only give rise to difficulties at estimating its prevalence [17, 22] but can also delay research of the most efficient treatment schemes.

2.2 Prevalence of resistant depression

In spite of pharmacological treatment advances in major depression, the final objective of achieving a sustained improvement continues to be insufficient [23]. It is estimated that about only 30–40% of patients achieve remission after the first attempt of treatment with antidepressants. In 3671 ambulatory patients treated with escitalopram, only 37% achieved remission [18]. Even after an appropriate sequence of treatments, 10–20% of the patients with major depression continue with significant symptoms for 2 years or more [24, 25]. The STAR*D study (sequenced treatment alternatives to relieve depression study) showed that accumulated remission after four treatment trials with antidepressants for 14 months was 67% [26]. Patients with chronic depression seem to have less opportunity for recovery [27] and tend to be more resistant to treatment [1, 28]. TRD is also associated to longer time of treatment and increased costs [29].

2.3 Antidepressant treatment resistance assessment scales and stratification systems

2.3.1 Antidepressant treatment assessment scales

From the multiple published assessment scales, three of them stand out in literature: the Antidepressant Treatment History Form [30], the Harvard Antidepressant Treatment History [31], and the Massachusetts General Hospital Antidepressant Treatment Response Questionnaire [6]. The clinician performs the former two; the latter is performed by the patient.

The Antidepressant Treatment History Form (ATHF; 1990; revised 1999) was originally designed to assess the efficacy of antidepressant treatment before ECT [30]. The scale has five treatment levels, which go from 0 (no treatment) to 5 (high antidepressant doses plus lithium or triiodothyronine (T3) for at least 4 weeks, including antipsychotics in patients with depression and psychotic symptoms. The scale has been modified and recently digitalized [32]. This scale has the disadvantage of not including pharmacological combination strategies or preferences on switching treatment [33]. The Antidepressant Treatment History Form has been empirically validated with the monitoring of prospective treatment [8, 33–35]. The original ATHF version has a good inter-rater reliability [3], and the digitalized version has an excellent inter-rater reliability as well, with another evaluator [32].

The Harvard Antidepressant Treatment History (HATH) allows to systematically assess the dose and duration of previous antidepressant medication trials. The patient identifies all the antidepressants taken from a list of all available once, a series of systematic questions over dose, duration, and response are asked to determine treatment response or resistance [31].

The Massachusetts General Hospital Antidepressant Treatment Response Questionnaire (ATRQ) is an auto-evaluating scale that defines an appropriate antidepressant treatment as optimal dosage during 6 weeks. This questionnaire provides operational criteria for adequate dosing of each antidepressant and has been used on multiple multicentric studies in TRD. In one study, it was found that MGH and ATRQ agree with the independent evaluations of clinical researchers on remote interviews [36].

2.3.2 Treatment resistant depression stratification systems

Systems may help predict the ulterior course of depression on the long-term and its response to treatment [1]. It is important to point out that all systems based on treatment administration have limitations; they were designed when therapeutic options available at the time were more limited, and despite their clinical usefulness, they have not been properly validated.

Four stratification systems stand out in literature: the Staging Method of Thase and Rush [4], the European Staging Method [5, 37], the Massachusetts General Hospital Staging model (MGH-s) [6], and The Maudsley Staging Model (MSM) [7].

Thase and Rush proposed five levels of resistance, in which patients are categorized according to the number and antidepressant class they have failed to respond, from the most frequently used to the least usual as MAOIs or ECT [4]. Not one degree of each therapeutic trial in terms of dose and duration is recorded; it assumes that the non-response to two antidepressant agents of different classes is more difficult to treat than the non-response to agents of the same group and that the change to an antidepressant of the same group is less effective. The later may be true for tricyclic antidepressants, but it is not so at switching between different serotonin reuptake inhibitors (SSRIs) [17]. This classification considers that the most effective antidepressants on order would be MAOIs, tricyclic antidepressants, and SSRIs, which has not been validated on different meta-analyses in antidepressant trials [17, 20]. It also faces the disadvantage of not including other treatments, such as drug combinations and psychotherapy, and does not provide prognostic information [38]. The Thase and Rush scale is easy to implement and provides an accessible strategy for clinicians to treat TRD patients. However, it has been widely criticized recently, since its predictive value over the course of treatment has not been systematically evaluated [8, 33, 34].

A European Staging Method (ESM) proposes the classification between non-responders, patients with TRD, and chronic resistant depression (CRD). Non-responders are defined as patients who fail to respond to a method of treatment. Patients are considered TRD if they show poor response to two treatment options with different classes of antidepressants at a proper dose over the span of 6–8 weeks. CRD is defined as a resistant or refractory episode that lasts for more than a year despite appropriate therapeutic interventions. This scale has the advantage of including the duration of the depressive episodes and does not suggest a hierarchy of antidepressants. Non-response is clearly defined as a reduction inferior to 50% on the score of the HAMD [39] or the Montgomery Asberg Depression Rating Scale (MADRS) [40] and the TRD stages correspond to the number of failed therapeutic trials. It is assumed that patients with failure to respond to two agents of different classes would be more resistant than those who do not respond to two drugs of the same group and indirectly implies that switching to a drug from the same class is less effective [6]. It should be noted that, in this classification, the differences between TRD and CRD are arbitrary [8]. ESM does not establish that two or more attempts with failed antidepressants imply a higher level of TRD, in contrast with the publications that associate the number of changes with poor response to treatment [17, 18]. Furthermore, CRD does not consider non-pharmacological measures such as ECT or psychotherapy. To date, there are no studies that prove the predictive utility or reliability of the scale.

The Massachusetts General Hospital Staging model (MGH-s) was published for the first time by Fava [6] based on the scale by Thase and Rush. The MGH-s considers dosage optimization and separately prolonging the duration of treatment, as well as an operational criterion for minimal dose and duration of treatment. It includes measures for titration and combinations and does not rank antidepressant classes [41] or an implied preference between them or a change to the same group of drugs. The MGH-s considers the number of failed treatments and the intensity and optimization of each attempt and generates a continuous variable that reflects the degree of resistance to antidepressants. MGH-s generates a continuous score that reflects the level of resistance. However, this score is randomly given [8]. Dosage optimization and duration are considered equal to increase or combination, which does not seem to be backed up on literature [42–44]. Finally, the higher score given to ECT is not sufficiently explained [7, 45].

A study published a comparison between the MGH-s and the Thase and Rush Staging Method on a sample of 115 ambulatory patients with major depression. All results showed that both models have a high correlation, but the multivariable analysis demonstrated that the MGH-s had a better prediction for non-remission [45].

Fedaku et al. [7] published The Maudsley Staging Model (MSM) method of stratification, in which the TDR score varies from 3 to 15. TRD stages are shown in three categories: mild (scores 3–6), moderate (scores 7–10), and severe (scores 11–15). It incorporates the duration and severity of the depressive episode. MSM considers class switching between different antidepressant groups, and between the same group has the same score. The scale is easy to use and may be employed as a tridimensional model regarding duration, severity, and treatment. It has been criticized, however, that disease duration is arbitrary and does not include the number of titrating attempts. Empiric value and inter-rate reliability was proven with prospective data obtained from the notes of 88 patients on a TRD specialized unit and follow-up of 62 patients in this group for a medium of 29.5 months [7].

2.4 Resistant depression treatment general principles

Qualitative and quantitative assessment of depressive symptoms with evaluation scales on each visit, assessment tool employment, and watching over adverse effects should be a routine practice in the approach to the patient with major depressive disorder, and even more so with the TRD patient. Furthermore, it is recommended to evaluate psychosocial performance, quality of life, treatment compliance and tolerance, and provide 24-h assistance [46]. It is important to encourage patients not to abandon treatment or medical attention despite of not perceiving any results. A good relationship between the clinician and the patient is also important to guarantee treatment compliance [15]. Finally, the role of psycho-education for the patients and their relatives should not be forgotten, as this includes sign and symptom identification, prognosis, suicide risk assessment, treatment options, sleep hygiene, impulse control, and sleep restriction among others. Behind restriction the initial management of depressive patients is usually done by primary care physicians or internists, but they should be referred to a mental health specialist if there is not an appropriate response to two or more treatments, as well when suicidal or homicidal ideation, psychotic or catatonic behavior are detected.

2.4.1 Treatment strategies

For patients with major depressive disorder who do not respond to initial treatment with an antidepressant, there are diverse management strategies [5, 14, 30, 47–50] which have been classified and arranged in three groups as follows: (1) optimization; (2) treatment switching (to a different antidepressant, psychotherapy, or ECT); (3) augmentation or adding other treatment to the one already in use, such as a different drug, psychotherapy, or ECT (**Table 1**). Regardless of the strategy, it is recommended always to use one strategy at a time to assess which is the most effective. We will review each one of them.

2.4.1.1 Optimization

Optimization consists of improving the current treatment, while supervising good tolerance. It should be noted that, in some studies with patients diagnosed as resistant and sent to specialized clinics, it has been reported that an important number of them did not receive an appropriate dose of the medication or had been taking it behind for a brief period of time [51]. This would represent a case of pseudo-resistance. Several studies show that it is important to treat a major depressive episode for 6–12 weeks before concluding non-remittance [6, 26, 52]. A study in

Strategy	Definition	Action
Optimization	Consists in improving the current treatment	Increase antidepressant's dosage Increase time exposure on treatment
Treatment switching	It is the act of suspending the current treatment and replacing it with other	Change of antidepressant Same classe of antidressant Different classe of antidepressant Switching to psychotherapy ECT
Augmentation	Consists of adding other treatments	A second antidepressant A second-generation antipsychotic Lithium Thyroid hormones Stimulants NMDA receptor acting drugs rTMS Psychotherapy

Table 1.
Treatment strategies for resistant depression.

1627 patients, where 67% of them received less than 4 weeks of treatment and did not show response to an antidepressant [53], did not find any difference between continuing the current treatment or changing to another antidepressant. This supports the importance of keeping the patients on an antidepressant treatment for an appropriate amount of time before changing it. On the other hand, multiple studies show that if patients have less than 25% reduction of symptoms after 4 weeks treatment, it could be indicated to switch to a different treatment strategy [54].

2.4.1.2 Treatment switching

Treatment switching is the act of suspending the current treatment and replacing it with a different pharmacologic or non-pharmacologic anti-depressive strategy. This includes using a different antidepressant, switching to psychotherapy, or ECT.

2.4.1.3 Changing antidepressants

It has been suggested that, in order to switch antidepressant medications, the current medication should be gradually discontinued while the new one is slowly introduced throughout 1–2 weeks and the dosage of the new antidepressant agent should be given at a corresponding amount to the one being discontinued. The clinician should be aware of increases of adverse effects and, in relation to SSRIs, the risk of serotonin syndrome. Some clinicians prefer to switch from an SSRI to another instantly, except when the patient has received fluoxetine, where the waiting time should be no less than 4 weeks before using another SSRI due to its long half-life.

For patients resistant to SSRIs, it has been suggested to switch to a selective noradrenaline and serotonin reuptake inhibitor (SNRI), atypical antidepressants, such as bupropion or mirtazapine, tricyclic antidepressants, or MAOIs. There are, however, few studies that compare switching to each one of these groups of drugs. In one meta-analysis that included four randomized studies with 1496 patients resistant to an SSRI, remission was evident in 24% of the patients who received another SSRI, and in 28% who were introduced to a different class of antidepressant such as bupropion, mirtazapine, or venlafaxine [55]. Regarding patients resistant to SSRI, many studies, including some meta-analyses, support changing to venlafaxine [17, 55]. A meta-analysis with 3375 patients with depression resistant to an SSRI showed that changing to another SSRI led to remission on 45% of the subjects, but 54% remitted when changing to venlafaxine [17]. Concerning atypical antidepressants, the few comparative studies available on TRD patients have not found differences respecting efficacy [18, 42]. In a group of patients resistant to paroxetine, a study that compared extended release venlafaxine (225 mg/day) and mirtazapine (45 mg/day) found remissions of 41 and 36% respectively [56]. In another study, 477 patients resistant to an SSRI treated for 14 weeks with bupropion SR (average dose 238 mg/day) or sertraline (average dose 136 mg/day) remission was achieved on 21 and 18% of the subjects, respectively [57]. An 8-week study that compared mirtazapine (45 mg/day) with paroxetine (20 mg/day) in 100 patients with TRD, remission was achieved in 36 and 47% with similar tolerance. Finally, a comparative study with mirtazapine (average dose 30 mg/day) and sertraline (average dose 120 mg/day) in 250 TRD patients, remission was similar (38 versus 28%, respectively) without statistical difference [58–60]. Nevertheless, there were more adverse effects with mirtazapine such as sedation, fatigue, weight gain, and xerostomia. In TRD patients, efficacy and tolerability of tricyclic antidepressants is comparable to that of atypical antidepressants and SSRIs [61]. Currently, tricyclic antidepressants have become the fourth or fifth line of treatment in TRD patients due to undesired adverse effects such as anticholinergic effects, cardiotoxicity, and lethal potential with overdose. The STAR*D study reported the fourth or fifth line of treatment in major depressive patients due to undesired adverse effects such as anticholinergic effects, cardiotoxicity, and lethal potential with overdose. In TRD patients, efficacy and tolerability of tricyclic antidepressants is comparable to that of atypical antidepressants and SSRIs. In the STAR*D study, an open 14-week trial in 235 patients compared nortriptyline (average dose 97 mg/day) with mirtazapine (average dose 42 mg/day) showing a comparable remission of 20 versus 12% and equal tolerance [62]. In a double-blind randomized study, 168 imipramine- or sertraline-resistant patients treated for 12 weeks were randomly assigned to the other treatment [63]. Remission was comparable (23% versus 32%) with more discontinuation with imipramine switching due to adverse effects (9 versus 0%). MAOIs are rarely used today, since they carry lethal potential by interacting with other drugs and food containing tyramine [64]. Nevertheless, changing to a MAOI may still be helpful for some TRD patients [17, 64]. A randomized trial with 46 imipramine-resistant patients who received phenelzine (45–90 mg/day) for 6 weeks and 22 phenelzine-resistant patients who were switched to imipramine (150–300 mg/day) reported a higher response on patients who received phenelzine rather than imipramine (67 versus 41%) [64]. For severely depressed patients with TRD, there is not enough evidence that indicates which kind of antidepressant is superior [65]. Tricyclic antidepressants may be preferred [66]. However, a meta-analysis of 25 randomized trials on 1377 hospitalized depressed patients who received tricyclic antidepressants or SSRIs showed that tricyclic antidepressant superiority over SSRIs was low with a higher rate of adverse effects [67].

2.4.1.4 Switching to psychotherapy

Changing from a pharmacologic approach to psychotherapy may be rejected by many TRD patients [68], but still is a reasonable approach. A 12-week trial with 122 patients who did not respond to citalopram and were randomized to cognitive behavioral therapy (CBT) or different antidepressants (bupropion, sertraline, or venlafaxine) [68] reported similar remission (25 and 28%). Another study with 140 patients who did not respond to a trial with nefazodone or CBT and then were switched to the other treatment [69] reported a comparable remission of 36 and 27%, respectively.

2.4.1.5 Electroconvulsive therapy

For patients with TRD with severe depression, ECT continues to be the therapy of choice [28, 66, 70–72]. The most important indications for ECT are persistence of suicidal ideation, suicide attempt, severe weight loss with malnutrition, dehydration, food or fluids rejection, and malignant catatonia. ECT is also indicated in cases of depression with psychotic symptoms and if there is previous history of response to this treatment. ECT has been shown superior to pharmacotherapy as shown by multiple meta-analyses and randomized studies [65]. A meta-analysis of 18 studies with 1144 patients that compared ECT with pharmacotherapy found that ECT was more effective [71]. ECT approach is recommended by many guidelines [66, 70, 72, 73]. ECT is not exempt of anesthetic risks, adverse effects, logistic problems, treatment rejection, and relapse.

2.4.1.6 Augmentation

Augmentation consists of adding other treatment (pharmacologic or non-pharmacologic) to the current one [74]. A new drug, psychotherapy, or transcranial magnetic stimulation (TME) might be added. This approach has been widely used and studied; combination therapy with antipsychotics, lithium, or triiiodothyronine (T3) are generally well tolerated [52, 58, 75–79], while combination therapy of MAOI with other antidepressants may cause serotonin syndrome or hypertensive crisis [80]. Previous response, safety, comorbidities, ease of use, patient's preference, and costs are factors to consider while adding other drugs to the current treatment. TRD patients, who have had additions and do not respond in 6–12 weeks at the desired dose or do not tolerate the combination, should be switched to a second combination [58]. Some authors suggest discontinuation of the supplementary drug and addition of a new one progressively over 1–2 weeks [58].

2.4.1.7 Adding a second antidepressant

Concerning depression with partial response to monotherapy with antidepressants, a second drug is usually added. However, a meta-analysis of eight studies with 808 patients that did not respond to monotherapy and that compared antidepressant combination with monotherapy, found a similar improvement on both groups [81]. The most studied antidepressants are mirtazapine and bupropion.

Mirtazapine use as an augmentation drug on TRD patients is supported by the results of open and placebo-controlled studies [81, 82]. On the STAR*D study, mirtazapine was added to patients resistant to venlafaxine and was compared with switching to tranylcypromine (a MAOI). Both approaches had no different effects [83]. However, addition of mirtazapine to resistant patients requires additional studies to establish its efficacy.

Bupropion, a noradrenergic/dopaminergic reuptake inhibitor, was studied in TRD patients [84]. Bupropion has a good tolerability and low side effect profile, including few sexual side effects.

Buspirone, a serotonin (5-HT1A) receptor partial agonist, was studied in randomized, double-blind, placebo-controlled trials combined with an SSRI in patients with TRD [85]. Buspirone, at a dosage of 41 mg/day, was compared on the STAR*D study with Bupropion SR at 267 mg/day, with similar effectiveness [44]. As with mirtazapine, bupropion addition is a popular practice as an enhancing maneuver, but additional studies are needed to justify its use on TRD patients.

2.4.1.8 Second-generation antipsychotics

For second-generation antipsychotics in patients with TRD, the following order was suggested based on benefit and a lower rate of adverse effects: aripiprazole, quetiapine, risperidone, and less frequently ziprasidone or olanzapine [58, 77, 86, 87]. Also, the use of brexpiprazole has been suggested if aripiprazole generates akathisia [88, 89]. The analysis of 16 studies comparing the addition of aripiprazole, olanzapine, quetiapine, or risperidone with placebo on 3480 patients with non-psychotic depression who failed to at least one attempt with antidepressant monotherapy [90] showed improvement in 31% of the patients who received the additional drug (31%) versus placebo (17%). Discontinue due to adverse effects was higher with antipsychotics (9 versus 2%), 4% for aripiprazole, 12% for quetiapine, and 7% for risperidone [90]. In an open, randomized 12-week trial with 1522 patients who stayed severely depressed after treatment with an antidepressant [75], the subjects received three types of treatments: aripiprazole increase (target dose 5–15 mg/day), bupropion increase (target dose 300–400 mg/day), or switching to bupropion. Response (reduction equal or higher than 50% of depression) was greater with aripiprazole (74%) than increasing bupropion (66%) or switching to bupropion (62%). There were more adverse effects with aripiprazole, such as akathisia, somnolence, weight gain, and laboratory abnormalities, but patients experienced more anxiety with bupropion. A meta-analysis of 11 randomized trials on TRD patients (n > 3000) found that effectiveness of the augmentation of atypical antipsychotics might rise with the increase of the resistance [90]. For example, the augmentation may carry more benefit for patients that do not respond to three or four failed attempts compared with those who do not respond to one.

2.4.1.9 Lithium

Augmentation of treatment with lithium was reported for the first time by De Montigny by combining it with tricyclic antidepressants [91]. Thereafter, multiple studies have demonstrated its efficacy. A meta-analysis of 10 placebo, controlled studies showed that the addition of lithium at a dose to 600–900 mg/day (plasma levels higher than 0.4 mEq/L) was superior to placebo [78, 92]. A meta-analysis of nine trials with 237 patients comparing lithium versus placebo found a higher response with lithium [84]. Lithium was effective in the augmentation with first- and second-generation antidepressants attached to a possible benefit in reducing suicide risk. A meta-analysis of nine studies with 234 patients, where double-blind trials with lithium and placebo on TRD patients were included, showed a broad effectiveness with this approach [93]. The authors concluded that it should be given for no less than 7 days at dose of 600–800 mg/day [93]. An analysis of the literature reviewing 12 randomized studies on lithium augmentation of SSRIs or atypical antipsychotic drug therapy found no statistical difference that favors the use of one approach or the other [94].

2.4.1.10 Thyroid hormone

Thyroid hormone, in particular T3, has been used as an augmenting agent since the 1960s [95]. The usual dose of T3 in the form of liothyronine is 25–50 pg and with thyroxine (T4) is 150 pg. An initial meta-analysis with T3 showed effectiveness against placebo [79]. Subsequent studies, however, have shown limited evidence of its effectiveness. A meta-analysis with four randomized studies with 95 patients who did not respond to tricyclic antidepressants compared augmentation with T3 versus placebo or T4 showed response in 53% patients who received T3 but had not statistical difference with placebo [79]. However, T3 augmentation is not very popular in the UK nor in the USA [96].

2.4.1.11 Repetitive transcranial magnetic stimulation

Repetitive transcranial magnetic stimulation (rTMS) is a non-invasive technique in which a sequence of high-intensity magnetic pulses is used to stimulate cortical neurons to treat neuropsychiatric disorders including major depressive disorder

[97]. This technique may be ambulatory, can be added to the current antidepressant treatment, and has good tolerability. Initial systematic reviews on mixed populations of depressed patients that included non-resistant patients supported their use on TRD patients [98–103]. A meta-analysis of 24 trials that included 1092 patients who underwent rTMS and sham conditions showed rTMS was superior in clinical improvement of patients with TRD. The response and remissions were 25 and 17% and 9 and 6% for the rTMS and sham conditions, respectively [104]. Short duration rTMS (1–4 weeks) has an evident antidepressant effect on TRD patients and is well tolerated. Nevertheless, remission rates and responses with rTMS are low and it is unknown if there is a sustained effect. Not known is whether effects of TMS are sustained over time and its speed of onset [104].

2.4.1.12 Psychotherapy

Addition of CBT usually helps TRD patients, as demonstrated by multiple randomized studies [105–107]. In a randomized 1-year study with CBT (12–18 sessions), it was observed that remission occurred more on CBT group of patients (28%) than in patients who did not receive it (15%). In another study, depressive symptoms were minor on a self-report 40 months after patients received CBT [108]. A 12-week study compared citalopram plus 16-session CBT with citalopram plus additional pharmacological approaches such as bupropion or buspirone in 182 ambulatory patients resistant to citalopram [109]. The number of patients who achieved remission was similar (23 and 33%). A 12-week study that compared nefazodone treatment with 16- to 20-session CBT versus nefazodone alone on 446 ambulatory patients with chronic depression (medium of 8 years) showed remission in more patients undergoing the combination (48 versus 29%) [110]. In hospitalized patients with severe depression, combination therapy is a common practice and its effectiveness is clear. A 12-week study that compares CBT and pharmacotherapy with pharmacotherapy alone in 20 hospitalized patients with chronic depression found a similar improvement [111]. An observational 12-week study with CBT added to pharmacotherapy in 24 hospitalized patients with chronic depression [112] found a 46% reduction in depressive symptoms. In TRD patients, other types of psychotherapy such as group, family, or interpersonal therapy have not been well studied.

2.4.1.13 Other addition maneuvers

Several addition maneuvers have been employed in TRD patients, such as lamotrigine combination, stimulants like methylphenidate, modafinil, and pindolol among others. A meta-analysis which included 10 studies with 289 patients undergoing lamotrigine treatment concluded that this drug had little effect on non-bipolar TRD patients [113]. Controlled studies evaluating placebo versus methylphenidate have been negative despite its regular use [114]. Modafinil did not show a sustained effect in two controlled studies. However, a subsequent retrospective analysis suggests that modafinil may help TRD patients with fatigue and somnolence [115]. Pindolol, a non-selective beta-adrenergic antagonistic with effect in the 5-HT1A auto-receptor has shown negative results against placebo on TRD patients [116]. N-methyl-D-aspartate (NMDA) receptor acting drugs like memantine, ketamine, and riluzole have been studied. Controlled studies with memantine, an NMDA-receptor antagonist, have been negative [117]. Ketamine, an NMDA-receptor antagonist anesthetic, has shown positive antidepressant results in a controlled study against placebo in patients with TRD [118]. Riluzole, a putative glutamate release inhibitor used in the treatment of amyotrophic lateral sclerosis, did not show effectiveness on a controlled study to prevent relapse after ketamine use [119].

2.4.2 Studies comparing switching versus augmentation maneuvers

Multiple guidelines suggest how to use augmentation or switching maneuvers (The American Psychiatric Association, United Kingdom National Institute of Health and Clinical Excellence guidelines among others) [28, 66, 120, 121]. However, few randomized studies comparing the effectiveness of these maneuvers on TRD patients have been performed and most of them do not differ between those patients with little or no benefit from those who improve partially.

Various studies show that augmentation or switching maneuvers are equally efficient. Thus, multiple evaluations reviewing placebo-controlled randomized studies regarding augmentation and switching approaches show similar results [76]. The medium rate of remission with augmentation was 27% and switching was 22%, with response rates (reduction of 50% or more of the symptoms) of 38 and 40%, respectively [122]. A prospective study with citalopram on two groups of 269 patients who preferred augmentation with bupropion or buspirone to switching citalopram to bupropion, sertraline, or venlafaxine had a similar remission. A randomized study with 375 TRD patients, where several treatments were assigned, including five augmentations and two switching options [123, 124] showed similar results with 37 and 41% for each strategy. On the other hand, in a group with 1522 patients (85% men), almost 50% of them undergoing post-traumatic disorder, and who continued severely depressed after the first course of treatment with an antidepressant, almost all of them on psychotherapy, the augmentation approach with aripiprazole (5–15 mg/day) or bupropion (300–400 mg/day) was slightly superior to switching antidepressants to bupropion as monotherapy [75]. Remission was achieved in 29% of the patients with aripiprazole augmentation, 27% with bupropion augmentation, and 22% with switching to bupropion. Surveillance over 24 months of the remitted patients (n = 396) showed that approximately 25% of the patients in each group relapsed. There were more adverse effects in the aripiprazole group [75]. Other studies show that augmentation approach with aripiprazole may be more effective in women than in men [125].

With patients not tolerating the antidepressant dose, it is preferable to switch antidepressants. While there is evidence that suggests that augmentation is somehow superior to switching antidepressants, the decision should be discussed with the patient. Clinical criteria would be that patients who have had partial benefit from the initial antidepressant and have few adverse effects may prefer an augmentation approach and those with less improvement and more adverse effects might prefer switching medication. However, in patients resistant to a second treatment, there is no evidence that shows how many approaches should be done before considering change of treatment. Authors suggest 1–3 trials before switching [58, 74]. Changing medications has the advantage of achieving a better compliance to treatment than when more than one medication is used [126] adding a lower risk of adverse effects, pharmacologic interactions, and costs. A study evaluated 48 trials that included 6654 patients. A comparison was made between randomized studies, which compared 11 agents used on augmentation approaches: atypical antipsychotics (aripiprazole, olanzapine, quetiapine, and risperidone), antidepressants (bupropion, buspirone), lithium, thyroid hormone, methylphenidate, pindolol, and lamotrigine [87]. The studies analyzed were compared between them or placebo in patients with TRD and the proportion of patients who responded to treatment was defined as primary effectiveness. The analysis showed that primary effectiveness was higher with quetiapine, aripiprazole, thyroid hormone, and lithium in relation to placebo, but even higher for the former two in the sensibility analysis. There were no differences regarding discontinuation rate and adverse effects (acceptability) for these treatments [87]. Quetiapine, olanzapine, aripiprazole, and lithium were less well tolerated than placebo [87].

A randomized 8-week study on 140 TRD patients with paroxetine plus risperidone, paroxetine plus trazodone, and paroxetine plus thyroid hormone showed similar remission rates of 27, 43, and 38%, respectively [123]. A 6-week randomized open study that compared adding quetiapine (target dose 300 mg/day) with adding lithium (target plasma concentration from 0.6 to 1.2 mmol/L) in 450 resistant patients got a similar remission rate of 32 and 27%, respectively [127].

A meta-analysis with 48 randomized trials (n > 6000 depressed patients) in which efficiency of augmentation agents was evaluated using results from comparisons between drugs (on head to head trials), as well as indirect comparisons of the drugs through their relative effects with a common comparator (typically a placebo) [123]. The response (reduction equal or higher than 50%) or remission was more frequent when aripiprazole, lithium, olanzapine, quetiapine, risperidone, or thyroid hormone (T3 or T4) was added, compared to placebo; results from each one were comparable. Discontinuation due to adverse effects was higher with aripiprazole, lithium, olanzapine, and quetiapine than with placebo.

2.4.3 Promising new treatments

2.4.3.1 Acetylcholine receptor acting drugs

Medications that act on the cholinergic system seem promising in the treatment of TRD patients. Controlled studies versus placebo with intravenous scopolamine (a muscarinic antagonist) in TRD patients showed promising results [128]. Mecamylamine, a nAChR antagonist added to citalopram, was also superior to placebo [129]. Other drugs like mecamylamine, S-mecamylamine, and varenicline are currently in a preliminary stage of study in depressive patients [129, 130].

2.4.3.2 N-methyl-D-aspartate (NMDA) acting drugs

Ketamine, an NMDA-receptor antagonist, has shown antidepressant effects in TRD patients in a controlled study versus placebo [118]. However, ketamine, a dissociative anesthetic administration which complicates TRD patient treatment due to its route of administration (intravenous), requires hospitalization and consultation with an anesthesiologist. The rapid effects of ketamine usually disappear in 4–6 days. Also, it is possible that patients who improve on ketamine require a long-term course of maintenance. Ketamine has been given intranasal, or by sublingual delivery. Lapidus et al. [131] compared intranasal administration of ketamine 50 mg and placebo in 20 TRD patients. Patients improved at 24 h, but not at 72 h after administration. Recent studies are currently researching intranasal administration of esketamine, the S-enantiomer of racemic ketamine on TRD patients. Initial results are very promising [132]. If accepted, esketamine would enter the list of enhancement approaches for TRD patients.

Deep brain stimulation, vagus nerve stimulation, and neurosurgical lesions have also been evaluated in different studies as therapeutic options in highly resistant TRD patients [133].

2.5 Neurobiological aspects of resistant depression

Most antidepressants act by modulating serotonin, noradrenaline, and dopamine neurotransmission, but other neurotransmission routes seem to be involved such as cholinergic, glutamatergic, neuropeptides, and neuromodulators among others. The complex neurotransmission systems are prone to failure in the short- or long-term, blocking antidepressant action. Besides, different antidepressant treatments seem to exert action by different mechanisms modulating different cerebral regions [134]. Genetic variants may explain up to 42% of antidepressant response [135]. Genetic polymorphisms for cytochrome P-450 (CYP) enzymes may lead to a reduction on enzyme activity of the CYP2D6 or CYP3A4 variants, leading to intolerance to antidepressants on high plasmatic levels [136, 137]. Some patients are rapid metabolizers, resulting in low plasmatic levels at standard doses of antidepressants, leading to resistance. Evaluation of these genetic variants is accessible with pharmacogenetic studies of antidepressants. Other resistance genetic variants may be related to p-glycoprotein (p-gp), also known as the $ABCB_1$ drug multiresistance gene [138]. Besides this, other polymorphic variants have been associated with response to antidepressants. In the case of serotonin 2A gene (HTR2A), both coding and noncoding polimorphisms have been associated to low SSRIs response [139–141]. Furthermore, single nucleotid polymorphisms (SNPs) of the genes for brain-derived neurotrophic factor (BDNF) [142, 143], the norepinephrine transporter [144], tryptophan hydroxylase 2 [145, 146], corticotrophin releasing hormone receptor 1 [147], the glucocorticoid receptor [148, 149], and the common promoter polymorphism of the serotonin transporter gene [150–155] have been associated with low SSRI response.

It has been published that the activation of the immune system and neuroinflammation represent a primary event in the pathophysiology of TRD [156–158] and that the effect of NSAID may increase the effect of antidepressants [159].

Finally, the catecholaminergic hypothesis of depression [160, 161], which associates depression with low levels of neurotransmitters, was accepted to explain not only the neurobiochemistry of depression, but also the effect of antidepressant drugs. This hypothesis postulates that, in depression, the function of the dopamine, noradrenaline, and indolamine serotonin monoamines is decreased. In support of this, different studies have shown changes in plasma, urine, and cerebrospinal fluid concentrations of these neurotransmitters and their metabolites, changes in the density of neuroreceptors in platelets and neurons, flattened curves in neuroendocrine challenges and also early relapses with the blockade of restriction enzymes for neurotransmitter synthesis in patients who had achieved depression remission with antidepressant treatment [162]. The existence of subtypes of depression, where noradrenergic, serotoninergic, or dopaminergic negative balance is predominant, has been also postulated. Patients with these subtypes of depression hypothetically would respond better to antidepressant drugs with noradrenergic, serotoninergic and dopaminergic effects. Unfortunately, clinical studies on the effect of antidepressants with different mechanisms of action show contradicting results, and today there are not clear clinical or biological parameters to predict the results of different antidepressant treatments [163]. It should be noted that any theory about the cause of TRD would be simplistic including that the deficit of a single neurotransmitter, genetic, or immune system and neuroinflammation responses would be present in most TRD patients. However, knowing if there are groups of patients that may respond better to drugs with different mechanisms of action continues to be important for the treatment of patients with TRD [164].

It has been suggested that, in the selection of an antidepressant drug, the clinician must observe the overall response of the patient with major depression [165]. Also, in the selection of an antidepressant drug, the clinician must observe the possible relationship between the drug's biochemical effect and its effects on specific symptoms but also on adverse events. This became more relevant when a drug or group of drugs have failed to improve the patient and a new one has to be supplied, when adverse events force treatment change or when augmentation or change of antidepressant treatment is considered.

3. Conclusions

Once resistance to treatment with two drugs with different action mechanisms has been established, the next best therapeutic decision is *terra ignota* because there is not enough scientific information available to validate which steps are to follow: whether change treatment, adding an antidepressant, "buster therapies" like addition of lithium, thyroid hormone or stimulants, add atypical antipsychotics, rTMS or employment of newly treatments such as ketamine, or ECT. In the evaluation stages for the treatment of a patient with TRD it is important to make an evaluation and reassessment of the case. This includes confirming the diagnosis of major depressive disorder, making the differential diagnoses of bipolar depression or other forms of resistant depression such as secondary to other medical issues, drugs, etc. Medical and psychiatric comorbidities, as well as depression severity should be assessed. Also, a detailed clinical history on antidepressant use should be performed. The application of diagnostic tools or evaluation scales is relevant.

Despite of its importance and frequency, there is no consensus over what TRD is. Advances have been made over assessment tools to evaluate resistance to treatment. However, there is no consensus over which is the best stratification system for TRD. There is a lack of research that validates which treatment approaches may be more effective and which ones should be used in the different stages in the management of a resistant patient. Unfortunately, advances over neurobiology of depression cannot be transferred yet to a clinical level to help the physician choose the best treatment for a patient with major depression and even less so for a TRD patient [163, 164]. In patients who have an inadequate response to the first line of treatment, the clinician has many options to change the treatment, but if the second approach fails, other approaches seem to be equally effective in according to what is published on the literature and there are no clear guidelines that support one or the other. This outlook is discouraging for patients and physicians who are on trial and error until they find something that helps the patient. Future research on TRD patients should be centered on neurobiological factors involved in the development of the resistance including pharmacogenetics. Without the development of techniques that help us predict which factors are related to this phenomenon, treatment of TRD patients will continue to be insufficient.

Acknowledgements

The author wishes to thank the Department of Psychiatry of the University Hospital UANL and the INFOSAME for its support in the preparation of this manuscript.

Conflict of interest

Dr. Jose Alfonso Ontiveros has received research grants from AstraZeneca, Glaxo Smith Kline, Eli Lilly, Servier, Wyeth, Lundbeck, Janssen-Cilag, Pfiser, and Sunovion.

Author details

Jose Alfonso Ontiveros
Department of Psychiatry, Autonomous University of Nuevo Leon, Monterrey, Mexico

*Address all correspondence to: ontiverosalf@gmail.com

References

[1] Crown WH, Finkelstein S, Berndt ER, Ling D, Poret AW, Rush AJ, et al. The impact of treatment-resistant depression on healthcare utilization and cost. The Journal of Clinical Psychiatry. 2002;**63**(11):963-971

[2] Berlim MT, Turecki G. What is the meaning of treatment resistant/refractory major depression (TRD)? A systematic review of current randomized trials. European Neuropsychopharmacology. 2007;**17**(11):696-707

[3] Sackeim HA, Prudic J, Devanand DP, Decina P, Kerr B, Malitz S. The impact of medication resistance and continuation pharmacotherapy on relapse following response to electroconvulsive therapy in major depression. Journal of Clinical Psychopharmacology. 1990;**10**(2):96-104

[4] Thase ME, Rush AJ. When at first you don't succeed: Sequential strategies for antidepressant nonresponders. The Journal of Clinical Psychiatry. 1997;**58**(Suppl 13):23-29

[5] Souery D, Amsterdam J, de Montigny C, Lecrubier Y, Montgomery S, Lipp O, et al. Treatment resistant depression: methodological overview and operational criteria. European Neuropsychopharmacology. 1999;**9**(1-2):83-91

[6] Fava M. Diagnosis and definition of treatment-resistant depression. Biological Psychiatry. 2003;**53**(8):649-659

[7] Fekadu A, Wooderson S, Donaldson C, Markopoulou K, Masterson B, Poon L, et al. A multidimensional tool to quantify treatment resistance in depression: The Maudsley staging method. The Journal of Clinical Psychiatry. 2009;**70**(2):177-184

[8] Berlim MT, Turecki G. Definition, assessment, and staging of treatment-resistant refractory major depression: A review of current concepts and methods. Canadian Journal of Psychiatry. 2007;**52**(1):46-54

[9] Fawcett J, Kravitz HM. Treatment refractory depression. In: Schatzberg AF, editor. Common Treatment Problems in Depression. Washington DC: American Psychiatric Press; 1985. pp. 2-27

[10] Lehmann HE. Therapy-resistant depressions—A clinical classification. Pharmakopsychiatrie, Neuro-Psychopharmakologie. 1974;**7**(3):156-163

[11] Fava M, Davidson KG. Definition and epidemiology of treatment-resistant depression. The Psychiatric Clinics of North America. 1996; **19**:179-200

[12] Trivedi MH, Rush AJ, Wisniewski SR, Nierenberg AA, Warden D, Ritz L, et al. Evaluation of outcomes with citalopram for depression using measurement-based care in STAR*D: Implications for clinical practice. The American Journal of Psychiatry. 2006;**163**(1):28-40

[13] Vergouwen AC, Bakker A, Katon WJ, Verheij TJ, Koerselman F. Improving adherence to antidepressants: A systematic review of interventions. The Journal of Clinical Psychiatry. 2003;**64**(12):1415-1420

[14] O'Reardon JP, Amsterdam JD. Treatment-resistant depression: Progress and limitations. Psychiatric Annals. 1998;**28**:633-640

[15] Rush AJ, Thase ME, Dube S. Research issues in the study of difficult-to-treat depression. Biological Psychiatry. 2003;**53**:743-53.17

[16] Committee for Medicinal Product for Human Use (CHMP). Concept Paper on the Need for Revision of Note for Guidance on Clinical Investigation of Medicinal Products in the Treatment of Depression with regard to Treatment Resistant Depression; European Medicines Agency. 2009. pp. 1-4. Available from: https://www.ema.europa.eu/en/documents/scientific-guideline/concept-paper-need-revision-note-guidance-clinical-investigation-medicinal-products-treatment_en-0.pdf

[17] Ruhe HG, Huyser J, Swinkels JA, Schene AH. Switching antidepressants after a first selective serotonin reuptake inhibitor in major depressive disorder: A systematic review. The Journal of Clinical Psychiatry. 2006;**67**(12):1836-1855

[18] Rush AJ, Trivedi MH, Wisniewski SR, Nierenberg AA, Stewart JW, Warden D, et al. Acute and longer-term outcomes in depressed outpatients requiring one or several treatment steps: A STAR*D report. The American Journal of Psychiatry. 2006;**163**(11):1905-1917

[19] O'Reardon JP, Amsterdam JD. Overview of treatment-resistant depression and its management. In: Amsterdam JD, Hornig M, Nierenberg AA, editors. Treatment-Resistant mood disorders. New York (NY): Cambridge University Press; 2001. pp. 30-45

[20] O'Reardon JP, Brunswick DJ, Amsterdam JD. Treatment-resistant depression in the age of serotonin: Evolving strategies. Current Opinion in Psychiatry. 2000;**13**:93-98

[21] Henricus G, Ruhé HG, Van Rooijen G, Spijker J, Peeters F, Schene A. Staging methods for treatment resistant depression. A systematic review. Journal of Affective Disorders. 2012;**137**:35-45

[22] Nemeroff CB. Prevalence and management of treatment-resistant depression. The Journal of Clinical Psychiatry. 2007;**68**(Suppl 8):17-25

[23] Trivedi MH, Kleiber BA. Using treatment algorithms for the affective management of treatment-resistant depression. Journal of Clinical Psychiatry. 2001;**62**(Suppl 18):25-29

[24] Keitner GI, Ryan CE, Solomon DA. Realistic expectations and a disease management model for depressed patients with persistent symptoms. The Journal of Clinical Psychiatry. 2006;**67**(9):1412-1421

[25] Keller MB, Shapiro RW, Lavori PW, Wolfe N. Recovery in major depressive disorder: Analysis with the life table and regression models. Archives of General Psychiatry. 1982;**39**(8):905-910

[26] Rush AJ. STAR*D: What have we learned? The American Journal of Psychiatry. 2007;**164**:201

[27] Mueller TI, Keller MB, Leon AC, Solomon DA, Shea MT, Coryell W, et al. Recovery after 5 years of unremitting major depressive disorder. Archives of General Psychiatry. 1996;**53**(9):794-799

[28] Malhi GS, Adams D, Porter R, et al. Clinical practice recommendations for depression. Acta Psychiatrica Scandinavica. Supplementum. 2009;(439):8-26

[29] Ustün TB, Kessler RC. Global burden of depressive disorders: The issue of duration. The British Journal of Psychiatry. 2002;**181**:181-183

[30] Sackeim HA. The definition and meaning of treatment-resistant depression. The Journal of Clinical Psychiatry. 2001;**62**(Suppl 16):10-17

[31] Nierenberg AA, Keck P, Samson J, Rothschild AJ, Schatzberg AF. Methodological considerations for the study of treatment-resistant depression.

In: Amsterdam JD, editor. Refractory Depression. New York (NY): Raven Press; 1991. pp. 1-12

[32] Oquendo MA, Baca-Garcia E, Kartachov A, Khait V, Campbell CE, Richards M, et al. A computer algorithm for calculating the adequacy of antidepressant treatment in unipolar and bipolar depression. The Journal of Clinical Psychiatry. 2003;**64**(7):825-833

[33] Ruhé HG, van Rooijen G, Spijker J, Peeters FPML, Schene AH. Staging methods for treatment resistant depression. A systematic review. Journal of Affective Disorders. 2012;**137**(1-3):35-45

[34] Bird D, Haddad PM, Dursun SM. An overview of the definition and management of treatment-resistant depression. Klinik Psikofarmakoloji Bülteni. 2002;**12**:92-101

[35] Fagiolini A, Kupfer DJ. Is treatment-resistant depression a unique subtype of depression? Biological Psychiatry. 2003;**53**:640-648

[36] Chandler GM, Iosifescu D, Pollack M, Targum S, Fava M. Validation of the Massachusetts General Hospital Antidepressant Treatment History Questionnaire (ATRQ). CNS Neuroscience and Therapeutics. 2010;**16**:322-325. DOI: 10.1111/j.1755-5949.2009.00102.x

[37] Souery D, Lipp O, Massat I, Mendlewicz J. The characterization and definition of treatment-resistant mood disorders. In: Amsterdam JD, Hornig M, Nierenberg AA, editors. Treatment-Resistant Mood Disorders. New York (NY): Cambridge University Press; 2001. pp. 30-45

[38] Souery D, Van der Auwera K. The multiple facets of treatment-resistant depression. CNS Spectrums. 2004;**9**(11):803-807

[39] Hamilton M. A rating scale for depression. Journal of Neurology, Neurosurgery, and Psychiatry. 1960;**23**:56-61

[40] Montgomery SA, Asberg M. A new depression scale designed to be sensitive to change. The British Journal of Psychiatry. 1979;**1979**:134, 382-389

[41] Souery D, Papakostas GI, Trivedi MH. Treatment-resistant depression. The Journal of Clinical Psychiatry. 2006;**67**(Suppl 6):16-22

[42] Ruhe HG, Huyser J, Swinkels JA, Schene AH. Dose escalation for insufficient response to standard-dose selective serotonin reuptake inhibitors in major depressive disorder: Systematic review. The British Journal of Psychiatry. 2006;**189**:309-316

[43] Ruhe HG, Booij J, Weert HCV, Reitsma JB, Franssen EJF, Michel MC, et al. Evidence why dose-escalation of paroxetine in major depressive disorder is not effective: A 6-week, randomized-controlled trial with assessment of serotonin transporter occupancy. Neuropsychopharmacology. 2009;**34**:999-1010

[44] Trivedi MH, Fava M, Wisniewski SR, Thase ME, Quitkin F, Warden D, et al. Medication augmentation after the failure of SSRIs for depression. The New England Journal of Medicine. 2006;**354**(12):1243-1252

[45] Petersen T, Papakostas GI, Posternak MA, Kant A, Guyker WM, Iosifescu DV, et al. Empirical testing of two models for staging antidepressant treatment resistance. Journal of Clinical Psychopharmacology. 2005;**25**(4):336-341

[46] Keller MB. Issues in treatment-resistant depression. The Journal of Clinical Psychiatry. 2005;**66**:5-12

[47] Berman RM, Narasimhan M, Charney DS. Treatment-refractory

depression: Definitions and characteristics. Depression and Anxiety. 1997;**5**:154-164

[48] Sharan P, Saxena S. Treatment-resistant depression: Clinical significance, concept and management. National Medical Journal of India. 1998;**11**:69-79

[49] Shelton RC et al. Therapeutic options for treatment-resistant depression. CNS Drugs. 2010;**24**(2):131-161

[50] Kornstein SG, Schneider RK. Clinical features of treatment-resistant depression. The Journal of Clinical Psychiatry. 2001;**62**(Suppl 16):18-25

[51] Hirschfeld RM, Keller MB, Panico S, et al. The National Depressive and Manic-Depressive Association consensus statement on the under-treatment of depression. JAMA. 1997;**277**:333-340

[52] Papakostas GI. Managing partial response or nonresponse: Switching, augmentation, and combination strategies for major depressive disorder. The Journal of Clinical Psychiatry. 2009;**70**(Suppl 6):16

[53] Bschor T, Kern H, Henssler J, Baethge C. Switching the antidepressant after nonresponse in adults with major depression: A systematic literature search and meta-analysis. The Journal of Clinical Psychiatry. 2018;**79**(1):16r10749. DOI: 10.4088/JCP.16r10749

[54] Kudlow PA, McIntyre RS, Lam RW. Early switching strategies in antidepressant non-responders: Current evidence and future research directions. CNS Drugs. 2014;**28**:601

[55] Papakostas GI, Fava M, Thase ME. Treatment of SSRI-resistant depression: A meta-analysis comparing within-versus across-class switches. Biological Psychiatry. 2008;**63**:699

[56] Gaynes BN, Dusetzina SB, Ellis AR, et al. Treating depression after initial treatment failure: Directly comparing switch and augmenting strategies in STAR*D. Journal of Clinical Psychopharmacology. 2012;**32**:114

[57] Rush AJ, Trivedi MH, Wisniewski SR, et al. Bupropion-SR, sertraline, or venlafaxine-XR after failure of SSRIs for depression. The New England Journal of Medicine. 2006;**354**:1231

[58] Connolly KR, Thase ME. If at first you don't succeed: A review of the evidence for antidepressant augmentation, combination and switching strategies. Drugs. 2011;**71**:43

[59] Thase ME, Kremer C, Rodrigues H. Mirtazapine versus sertraline after SSRI non-response. European Neuropsychopharmacology. 2001;**11**(3):S342

[60] Thase ME. Mirtazapine vs. sertraline in SSRI TRD; Symposium abstracts: The International Society for Affective Disorders (ISAD) - 2nd Biennial Conference - Cancun, Mexico 5th - 10th March 2004. Journal of Affective Disorders. 2004;**78**(Suppl):S49

[61] Hirschfeld RM, Montgomery SA, Aguglia E, et al. Partial response and nonresponse to antidepressant therapy: Current approaches and treatment options. The Journal of Clinical Psychiatry. 2002;**63**:826

[62] Fava M, Rush AJ, Wisniewski SR, et al. A comparison of mirtazapine and nortriptyline following two consecutive failed medication treatments for depressed outpatients: A STAR*D report. The American Journal of Psychiatry. 2006;**163**:1161

[63] Thase ME, Rush AJ, Howland RH, et al. Double-blind switch study of imipramine or sertraline treatment of antidepressant-resistant chronic

depression. Archives of General Psychiatry. 2002;**59**:233

[64] Thase ME. The role of monoamine oxidase inhibitors in depression treatment guidelines. The Journal of Clinical Psychiatry. 2012;**73**(Suppl 1):10

[65] Fekadu A, Rane LJ, Wooderson SC, et al. Prediction of longer-term outcome of treatment-resistant depression in tertiary care. The British Journal of Psychiatry. 2012;**201**:369

[66] Anderson IM, Ferrier IN, Baldwin RC, et al. Evidence-based guidelines for treating depressive disorders with antidepressants: A revision of the 2000 British Association for Psychopharmacology guidelines. Journal of Psychopharmacology. 2008;**22**:343

[67] Anderson IM. SSRIS versus tricyclic antidepressants in depressed inpatients: A meta-analysis of efficacy and tolerability. Depression and Anxiety. 1998;**7**(Suppl 1):11

[68] Wisniewski SR, Fava M, Trivedi MH, et al. Acceptability of second-step treatments to depressed outpatients: A STAR*D report. The American Journal of Psychiatry. 2007;**164**:753

[69] Schatzberg AF, Rush AJ, Arnow BA, et al. Chronic depression: Medication (nefazodone) or psychotherapy (CBASP) is effective when the other is not. Archives of General Psychiatry. 2005;**62**:513

[70] Kennedy SH, Milev R, Giacobbe P, et al. Canadian Network for Mood and Anxiety Treatments (CANMAT) Clinical guidelines for the management of major depressive disorder in adults. IV. Neurostimulation therapies. Journal of Affective Disorders. 2009;**117**(Suppl 1):S44

[71] UK ECT Review Group. Efficacy and safety of electroconvulsive therapy in depressive disorders: A systematic review and meta-analysis. Lancet. 2003;**361**:799

[72] American Psychiatric Association. Practice guideline for the treatment of patients with major depressive disorder. 3rd ed. American Journal of Psychiatry. 2010;**167**(Supplement):1. Available from: http://psychiatryonline.org/guidelines.aspx [Accessed: April 17, 2012]

[73] Trangle M, Dieperink B, Gabert T, et al. Institute for Clinical Systems Improvement. Major Depression in Adults in Primary Care. Updated May 2012. Available from: http://www.icsi.org/depression_5/depression__major__in_adults_in_primary_care_3.html [Accessed: December 12, 2012]

[74] Thase ME. Augmentation strategies for depression: History and concepts. CNS Spectrums. 2007;**12**:3

[75] Mohamed S, Johnson GR, Chen P, et al. Effect of antidepressant switching vs augmentation on remission among patients with major depressive disorder unresponsive to antidepressant treatment: The VAST-D randomized clinical trial. JAMA. 2017;**318**:132

[76] Santaguida P, MacQueen G, Keshavarz H, et al. Treatment for Depression After Unsatisfactory Response to SSRIs. Comparative Effectiveness Review No. 62 (Prepared by McMaster University Evidence-based Practice Center under Contract No. HHSA 290 2007 10060 I). AHRQ Publication No. 12-EHC050-EF. Rockville, MD: Agency for Healthcare Research and Quality; 2012. Available from: www.ahrq.gov/clinic/epcix.htm

[77] Nelson JC, Papakostas GI. Atypical antipsychotic augmentation in major depressive disorder: A meta-analysis of placebo-controlled randomized trials. The American Journal of Psychiatry. 2009;**166**:980

[78] Crossley NA, Bauer M. Acceleration and augmentation of antidepressants with lithium for depressive disorders: Two meta-analyses of randomized, placebo-controlled trials. The Journal of Clinical Psychiatry. 2007;**68**:935

[79] Aronson R, Offman HJ, Joffe RT, Naylor CD. Triiodothyronine augmentation in the treatment of refractory depression. A meta-analysis. Archives of General Psychiatry. 1996;**53**:842

[80] Preskorn SH. Treatment options for the patient who does not respond well to initial antidepressant therapy. Journal of Psychiatric Practice. 2009;**15**:202

[81] Henssler J, Bschor T, Baethge C. Combining antidepressants in acute treatment of depression: A meta-analysis of 38 studies including 4511 patients. Canadian Journal of Psychiatry. 2016;**61**:29

[82] Carpenter LL, Yasmin S, Price LH. A double-blind, placebo-controlled study of antidepressant augmentation with mirtazapine. Biological Psychiatry. 2002;**51**(2):183-188

[83] McGrath PJ, Stewart JW, Fava M, Trivedi MH, Wisniewski SR, Nierenberg AA, et al. Tranylcypromine versus venlafaxine plus mirtazapine following three failed antidepressant medication trials for depression: A STAR*D report. The American Journal of Psychiatry. 2006;**163**(9):1531-1541. Quiz 666.31

[84] Bodkin JA, Lasser RA, Wines JD Jr, et al. Combining serotonin reuptake inhibitors and bupropion in partial responders to antidepressant monotherapy. The Journal of Clinical Psychiatry. 1997;**58**(4):137-145

[85] Landen M, Bjorling G, Agren H, Fahlen T. A randomized, double-blind, placebo-controlled trial of buspirone in combination with an SSRI in patients with treatment-refractory depression. The Journal of Clinical Psychiatry. 1988;**59**(12):664-668

[86] Philip NS, Carpenter LL, Tyrka AR, Price LH. Depression: A re-examination for the modern era. Expert Opinion on Pharmacotherapy. 2010;**11**(5):709-722

[87] Zhou X, Ravindran AV, Qin B, et al. Comparative efficacy, acceptability, and tolerability of augmentation agents in treatment-resistant depression: Systematic review and network meta-analysis. The Journal of Clinical Psychiatry. 2015;**76**(4):487-498

[88] Thase ME, Youakim JM, Skuban A, et al. Adjunctive brexpiprazole 1 and 3 mg for patients with major depressive disorder following inadequate response to antidepressants: A phase 3, randomized, double-blind study. The Journal of Clinical Psychiatry. 2015;**76**:1232

[89] Thase ME, Youakim JM, Skuban A, et al. Efficacy and safety of adjunctive brexpiprazole 2 mg in major depressive disorder: A phase 3, randomized, placebo-controlled study in patients with inadequate response to antidepressants. The Journal of Clinical Psychiatry. 2015;**76**:1224

[90] Wang HR, Woo YS, Ahn HS, et al. Can atypical antipsychotic augmentation reduce subsequent treatment failure more effectively among depressed patients with a higher degree of treatment resistance? A meta-analysis of randomized controlled trials. The International Journal of Neuropsychopharmacology. 2015;**18**:pyv023. Available from: https://www.ncbi.nlm.nih.gov/pmc/articles/PMC4571632/

[91] De Montigny C, Grunberg F, Mayer A, Deschenes JP. Lithium induces rapid relief of depression in tricyclic antidepressant drug non-responders. The British Journal of Psychiatry. 1981;**138**:252-256

[92] Nelson JC, Baumann P, Delucchi K, et al. A systematic review and meta-analysis of lithium augmentation of tricyclic and second generation antidepressants in major depression. Journal of Affective Disorders. 2014;**168**:269

[93] Bauer M, Döpfmer S. Lithium augmentation in treatment-resistant depression: Meta-analysis of placebo-controlled studies. Journal of Clinical Psychopharmacology. 1999;**19**(5):427-434

[94] Edwards SJ, Hamilton V, Nherera L, Trevor N. Lithium or an atypical antipsychotic drug in the management of treatment-resistant depression: A systematic review and economic evaluation. Health Technology Assessment. 2013;**17**(54):1-190

[95] Prange AJ Jr, Wilson IC, Rabon AM, Lipton MA. Enhancement of imipramine antidepressant activity by thyroid hormone. The American Journal of Psychiatry. 1969;**126**:457

[96] Dorling CM. Antidepressant augmentation and combinations. Psychiatric Clinics of North America. 2000;**23**(4):743-755

[97] Eitan R, Lerer B. Nonpharmacological, somatic treatments of depression: Electroconvulsive therapy and novel brain stimulation modalities. Dialogues in Clinical Neuroscience. 2006;**8**(2):241-258

[98] McNamara B, Ray JL, Arthurs OJ, et al. Transcranial magnetic stimulation for depression and other psychiatric disorders. Psychological Medicine. 2001;**31**(7):1141-1146

[99] Holtzheimer PE, Russo J, Avery DH. A meta-analysis of repetitive transcranial magnetic stimulation in the treatment of depression. Psychopharmacology Bulletin. 2001;**35**(4):149-169

[100] Burt T, Lisanby SH, Sackeim HA. Neuropsychiatric applications of transcranial magnetic stimulation: A meta analysis. The International Journal of Neuropsychopharmacology. 2002;**5**(1):73-103

[101] Kozel FA, George MS. Meta-analysis of left prefrontal repetitive transcranial magnetic stimulation (rTMS) to treat depression. Journal of Psychiatric Practice. 2002;**8**(5):270-275

[102] Martin JL, Barbanoj MJ, Schlaepfer TE, et al. Repetitive transcranial magnetic stimulation for the treatment of depression. Systematic review and meta-analysis. The British Journal of Psychiatry. 2003;**182**:480-491

[103] Couturier JL. Efficacy of rapid-rate repetitive transcranial magnetic stimulation in the treatment of depression: A systematic review and meta-analysis. Journal of Psychiatry & Neuroscience. 2005;**30**(2):83-90

[104] Lam RW, Chan P, Wilkins-Ho M, Yatham LN. Repetitive transcranial magnetic stimulation for treatment-resistant depression: A systematic review and metaanalysis. Canadian Journal of Psychiatry. 2008;**53**(9):621-631

[105] Trivedi RB, Nieuwsma JA, Williams JW Jr. Examination of the utility of psychotherapy for patients with treatment resistant depression: A systematic review. Journal of General Internal Medicine. 2011;**26**:643

[106] Eisendrath SJ, Gillung E, Delucchi KL, et al. A randomized controlled trial of mindfulness-based cognitive therapy for treatment-resistant depression. Psychotherapy and Psychosomatics. 2016;**85**:99

[107] Watkins ER, Mullan E, Wingrove J. et al, Rumination-focused cognitive-behavioural therapy for residual depression: Phase II randomised

controlled trial. The British Journal of Psychiatry. 2011;**199**:317

[108] Wiles NJ, Thomas L, Turner N, et al. Long-term effectiveness and cost-effectiveness of cognitive behavioural therapy as an adjunct to pharmacotherapy for treatment-resistant depression in primary care: Follow-up of the CoBalT randomised controlled trial. Lancet Psychiatry. 2016;**3**:137

[109] Thase ME, Friedman ES, Biggs MM, et al. Cognitive therapy versus medication in augmentation and switch strategies as second-step treatments: A STAR*D report. The American Journal of Psychiatry. 2007;**164**:739

[110] Keller MB, McCullough JP, Klein DN, et al. A comparison of nefazodone, the cognitive behavioral-analysis system of psychotherapy, and their combination for the treatment of chronic depression. The New England Journal of Medicine. 2000;**342**:1462

[111] Barker WA, Scott J, Eccleston D. The Newcastle chronic depression study: Results of a treatment regime. International Clinical Psychopharmacology. 1987;**2**:261

[112] Scott J. Chronic depression: Can cognitive therapy succeed when other treatments fail? Behavioural Psychotherapy. 1992;**20**:25

[113] Thomas SP, Nandhra HS, Jayaraman A. Systematic review of lamotrigine augmentation of treatment resistant unipolar depression (TRD). Review published. Journal of Mental Health. 2010;**19**(2):168-175

[114] Ravindran AV, Kennedy SH, O'Donovan MC, Fallu A, Camacho F, Binder CE. Osmotic-release oral system methylphenidate augmentation of antidepressant monotherapy in major depressive disorder: Results of a double-blind, randomized, placebo-controlled trial. The Journal of Clinical Psychiatry. 2008;**69**(1):87-94

[115] Fava M, Thase ME, De Battista C. A multicenter, placebo-controlled study of modafinil augmentation in partial responders to selective serotonin reuptake inhibitors with persistent fatigue and sleepiness. The Journal of Clinical Psychiatry. 2005;**66**(1):85-93

[116] Sokolski KN, Conney JC, Brown BJ, De Met EM. Once-daily high-dose pindolol for SSRI-refractory depression. Psychiatry Research. 2004;**125**(2):81-86

[117] Zarate CA, Singh JB, Quiroz JA, De Jesus G, Denicoff KK, Luckenbaugh DA, et al. A double-blind, placebo-controlled study of memantine in the treatment of major depression. The American Journal of Psychiatry. 2006;**163**(1):153-155

[118] Zarate CA, Singh JB, Carlson PJ, Brutsche NE, Ameli R, Luckenbaugh DA, et al. A randomized trial of an N-methyl-D-aspartate antagonist in treatment-resistant major depression. Archives of General Psychiatry. 2006;**63**(8):856-864

[119] Mathew SJ, Murrough JW, Aan Het Rot M, Collins KA, Reich DL, Charney DS. Riluzole for relapse prevention following intravenous ketamine in treatment-resistant depression: A pilot randomized, placebo-controlled continuation trial. The International Journal of Neuropsychopharmacology. 2009;**17**:1-12

[120] Kennedy SH, Lam RW, McIntyre RS, et al. Canadian Network for Mood and Anxiety Treatments (CANMAT) 2016 Clinical guidelines for the management of adults with major depressive disorder: Section 3. Pharmacological treatments. Canadian Journal of Psychiatry. 2016;**61**:540

[121] Spijker J, Nolen WA. An algorithm for the pharmacological treatment

of depression. Acta Psychiatrica Scandinavica. 2010;**121**:180

[122] Gaynes BN, Lux L, Lloyd S, et al. Nonpharmacologic Interventions for Treatment-Resistant Depression in Adults. Comparative Effectiveness Review No. 33. AHRQ Publication No. 11-EHC056-EF. Rockville, MD: Agency for Healthcare Research and Quality; 2011. Available from: http://www.effectivehealthcare.ahrq.gov/ or 800-358-9295. PMID: 22091472

[123] Fang Y, Yuan C, Xu Y, et al. A pilot study of the efficacy and safety of paroxetine augmented with risperidone, valproate, buspirone, trazodone, or thyroid hormone in adult Chinese patients with treatment-resistant major depression. Journal of Clinical Psychopharmacology. 2011;**31**:638

[124] Fang Y, Yuan C, Xu Y, et al. Comparisons of the efficacy and tolerability of extended-release venlafaxine, mirtazapine, and paroxetine in treatment-resistant depression: A double-blind, randomized pilot study in a Chinese population. Journal of Clinical Psychopharmacology. 2010;**30**:357

[125] Thase ME, Trivedi MH, Nelson JC, et al. Examining the efficacy of adjunctive aripiprazole in major depressive disorder: A pooled analysis of 2 studies. The Primary Care Companion to The Journal of Clinical Psychiatry. 2008;**10**:440

[126] Osterberg L, Blaschke T. Adherence to medication. The New England Journal of Medicine. 2005;**353**:487

[127] Bauer M, Dell'osso L, Kasper S, et al. Extended-release quetiapine fumarate (quetiapine XR) monotherapy and quetiapine XR or lithium as add-on to antidepressants in patients with treatment-resistant major depressive disorder. Journal of Affective Disorders. 2013;**151**:209

[128] Drevets WC, Zarate CA Jr, Furey ML. Antidepressant effects of the muscarinic cholinergic receptor antagonist scopolamine: A review. Biological Psychiatry. 2013;**73**:1156-1163

[129] George TP, Sacco KA, Vessicchio JC, Weinberger AH, Shytle RD. Nicotinic antagonist augmentation of selective serotonin reuptake inhibitor-refractory major depressive disorder: A preliminary study. Journal of Clinical Psychopharmacology. 2008;**28**:340-344

[130] Furey ML, Drevets WC. Antidepressant efficacy of the antimuscarinic drug scopolamine: A randomized, placebo-controlled clinical trial. Archives of General Psychiatry. 2006;**63**(10):1121-1129

[131] Lapidus KA, Levitch CF, Perez AM, Brallier JW, Parides MK, Soleimani L, et al. A randomized controlled trial of intranasal ketamine in major depressive disorder. Biological Psychiatry. 2014;**76**:970-976

[132] Daly EJ, Singh JB, Fedgchin M, Cooper K, Lim P, Shelton RC, et al. Efficacy and safety of intranasal esketamine adjunctive to oral antidepressant therapy in treatment-resistant depression. A randomized clinical trial. JAMA Psychiatry. 2018;**75**(2):139-148

[133] Cusin C, Dougherty DD. Somatic therapies for treatment-resistant depression: ECT, TMS, VNS, DBS. Biology of Mood & Anxiety Disorders. 2012;**2**:14

[134] Fu CH, Williams SC, Cleare AJ, et al. Attenuation of the neural response to sad faces in major depression by antidepressant treatment: A prospective, event-related functional magnetic resonance imaging study. Archives of General Psychiatry. 2004;**61**:877-889

[135] Tansey KE, Guipponi M, Hu X, Domenici E, Lewis G, Malafosse A, et al. Contribution of common genetic variants to antidepressant response. Biological Psychiatry. 2013;**73**:679-682

[136] Binder EB, Holsboer F. Pharmacogenomics and antidepressant drugs. Annals of Medicine. 2006;**38**:82-94

[137] de Leon J, Armstrong SC, Cozza KL. Clinical guidelines for psychiatrists for the use of pharmacogenetic testing for CYP450 2D6 and CYP450 2C19. Psychosomatics. 2006;**47**:75-85

[138] Abaut AY, Chevanne F, Le Corre P. Oral bioavailability and intestinal secretion of amitriptyline: Role of P-glycoprotein? International Journal of Pharmaceutics. 2007;**330**:121-128

[139] Peters EJ, Slager SL, McGrath PJ, et al. Investigation of serotonin-related genes in antidepressant response. Molecular Psychiatry. 2004;**9**:879-889

[140] Choi MJ, Kang RH, Ham BJ, et al. Serotonin receptor 2A gene polymorphism (−1438A/G) and short-term treatment response to citalopram. Neuropsychobiology. 2005;**52**:155-162

[141] McMahon FJ, Buervenich S, Charney D, et al. Variation in the gene encoding the serotonin 2A receptor is associated with outcome of antidepressant treatment. American Journal of Human Genetics. 2006;**78**:804-814

[142] Calabrese F, van der Doelen RH, Guidotti G, Racagni G, Kozicz T, Homberg JR, et al. Exposure to early life stress regulates Bdnf expression in SERT mutant rats in ananatomically selective fashion. Journal of Neurochemistry. 2015;**132**:146-154

[143] Tsai SJ, Cheng CY, Yu YW, et al. Association study of a brain-derived neurotrophic-factor genetic polymorphism and major depressive disorders, symptomatology, and antidepressant response. American Journal of Medical Genetics. Part B, Neuropsychiatric Genetics. 2003;**123**:19-22

[144] Kirchheiner J, Grundemann D, Schomig E. Contribution of allelic variations in transporters to the phenotype of drug response. Journal of Psychopharmacology. 2006;**20**:27-32

[145] Serretti A, Zanardi R, Cusin C, et al. Tryptophan hydroxylase gene associated with paroxetine antidepressant activity. European Neuropsychopharmacology. 2001;**11**:375-380

[146] Serretti A, Cusin C, Rossini D, et al. Further evidence of a combined effect of SERTPR and TPH on SSRIs response in mood disorders. American Journal of Medical Genetics. Part B, Neuropsychiatric Genetics. 2004;**129**:36-40

[147] Reul J, Holsboer F. Corticotrophin-releasing factor receptor 1 and 2 in anxiety and depression. Current Opinion in Pharmacology. 2002;**2**(1):23-33

[148] Liu Z, Zhu F, Wang G, et al. Association study of corticotropin-releasing hormone receptor1 gene polymorphisms and antidepressant response in major depressive disorders. Neuroscience Letters. 2007;**414**:155-158

[149] Brouwer JP, Appelhof BC, van Rossum EF, et al. Prediction of treatment response by HPA-axis and glucocorticoid receptor polymorphisms in major depression. Psychoneuroendocrinology. 2006;**31**:1154-1163

[150] Zanardi R, Benedetti F, Di Bella D, et al. Efficacy of paroxetine in depression is influenced by a functional polymorphism within the promoter of

the serotonin transporter gene. Journal of Clinical Psychopharmacology. 2000;**20**:105-107

[151] Zanardi R, Serretti A, Rossini D, et al. Factors affecting fluvoxamine antidepressant activity: Influence of pindolol and 5-HTTLPR in delusional and nondelusional depression. Biological Psychiatry. 2001;**50**:323-330

[152] Serretti A, Benedetti F, Zanardi R, Smeraldi E. The influence of Serotonin Transporter Promoter Polymorphism (SERTPR) and other polymorphisms of the serotonin pathway on the efficacy of antidepressant treatments. Progress in Neuro-Psychopharmacology & Biological Psychiatry. 2005;**29**:1074-1084

[153] Kraft JB, Peters EJ, Slager SL, et al. Analysis of association between the serotonin transporter and antidepressant response in a large clinical sample. Biological Psychiatry. 2007;**61**:734-742

[154] Caspi A, Sugden K, Moffitt TE, Taylor A, Craig IW, Harrington H, et al. Influence of life stress on depression: Moderation by a polymorphism in the 5-HTT gene. Science. 2003;**301**(5631):386-389

[155] Mancama D, Kerwin RW. Role of pharmacogenomics in individualising treatment with SSRIs. CNS Drugs. 2003;**17**:143-151

[156] Carvalho LA, Torre JP, Papadopoulos AS, Poon L, Juruena MF, Markopoulou K, et al. Lack of clinical therapeutic benefit of antidepressants is associated overall activation of the inflammatory system. Journal of Affective Disorders. 2013;**148**:136-140

[157] Gennarelli M, Uher R, Breen G, Farmer A, Aitchison KJ, Craig IW, et al. Candidate genes expression profile associated with antidepressants response in the GENDEP study: Differentiating between baseline 'predictors' and longitudinal 'targets'. Neuropsychopharmacology. 2013;**38**:377-385

[158] Kiraly DD, Horn SR, Van Dam NT, Costi S, Schwartz J, Kim-Schulze S, et al. Altered peripheral immune profiles in treatment-resistant depression: Response to ketamine and prediction of treatment outcome. Translational Psychiatry. 2017;7:e1065

[159] Abbasi SH, Hosseini F, Modabbernia A, Ashrafi M, Akhondzadeh S. Effect of celecoxib add-on treatment on symptoms and serum IL-6 concentrations in patients with major depressive disorder: Randomized double-blind placebo-controlled study. Journal of Affective Disorders. 2012;**141**:308-314

[160] Green AI, Schatzberg AF. Obituary. Joseph J. Schildkraut, 1934-2006. Neuropsychopharmacology. 2007;**32**:1855-1856

[161] Schildkraut JJ. The catecholamine hypothesis of affective disorders: A review of supporting evidence. The American Journal of Psychiatry. 1965;**122**:509-522

[162] Humble M. Noradrenaline and serotonin reuptake inhibition as clinical principle: A review of antidepressant efficacy. Acta Psychiatrica Scandinavica. 2000;**101**(Suppl 402):28-36

[163] Ontiveros A. Response to serotonergic and noradrenergic antidepressants: A crossover study of fluoxetine and desipramine in patients with first major depression episode. Gaceta Médica de México. 2017;**153**(6):188-194

[164] Coplan JD, Gopinath S, Abdallah C. Neurobiological hypothesis of treatment-resistant depression—Mechanisms for selective serotonin reuptake inhibitor non-efficacy.

Frontiers in Behavioral Neuroscience. 2014;**8**:189. DOI: 10.3389/fnbeh.2014.00189. Published online: May 20. 2014. PMCID: PMC4033019. PMID: 24904340A

[165] Thase M, Connolly KR, Roy-Byrne PP, Solomon D. Unipolar Depression in Adults: Treatment of Resistant Depression. Waltham, MA: Wolters Kluwer Health; 2015

Section 3

Preclinical and Translational Studies

Chapter 4

Influences of Maternal Vulnerability and Antidepressant Treatment during Pregnancy on the Developing Offspring

Laura Staal and Jocelien DA Olivier

Abstract

Maternal vulnerability to adversity has long-term impact on the developing child. About 20% of the pregnant women suffer from affective disorders. Fetal exposure to maternal adversity may lead to detrimental consequences later in life. Maternal affective disorders are increasingly treated with antidepressants, especially selective serotonin reuptake inhibitors (SSRIs). However, the long-term consequences for the offspring after exposure to this medication are unclear. The interplay between maternal adversity and SSRI treatment has been under investigation and here we discuss how maternal adversity and SSRIs are able to shape offspring development. Specifically, we will discuss animal models addressing behavioral outcomes to understand how the prenatal environment influences the health of the developing child across the life span.

Keywords: maternal vulnerability, maternal depression, selective serotonin reuptake inhibitors, antidepressants, pregnancy, neurodevelopment

1. Introduction

Although pregnancy is often portrayed as a time of great joy, that is not the reality for all women. Depressive symptoms during pregnancy are not uncommon; in fact, 20% of women experience some depressive symptoms during any time of their pregnancy [1]. The number of women who suffer from major depression during pregnancy is estimated to be 4–8% [2, 3]. According to the DSM-5, this disorder is characterized by a depressed mood or loss of interest or pleasure in daily activities for more than 2 weeks. Depression is accompanied by impaired social, occupational, and educational functioning. Untreated antenatal depression, that is to say a depressive episode during pregnancy, may have a tremendous effect on the developing child [4].

Maternal vulnerabilities during pregnancy, such as depression, anxiety, or high stress levels due to other reasons, are associated with increased and continued activation of the hypothalamic-pituitary-adrenal (HPA) axis. The continued activation of the HPA axis in depressed patients causes an elevated stress response and increased cortisol levels [5]. About 40% of the cortisol passes through the placenta [6]. Consequently, increased cortisol levels are found in the urine and saliva of the infants of depressed mothers [7].

IntechOpen

Fetal exposure to increased maternal stress levels impacts the developing child. For example, high levels of maternal cortisol are associated with reduced neurological development [8] and altered cortisol responses of the unborn child to a stressor [9]. Furthermore, maternal vulnerabilities such as anxiety, depression, and elevated stress levels are associated with the increased fearful temperament and negative behavioral reactivity to novelty in infants [9, 10], and delayed cognitive and neuromotor development [11, 12] that persists into adolescence [13]. In addition, antenatal depression has also been linked with disturbed sleep patterns in infants [14] and in 18 and 30 months old children [15]. Furthermore, antenatal depression has been linked to reduced fetal growth [16, 17] and altered cardiovascular responses to stress [18].

Several studies have looked into the effects of maternal vulnerability on the behavioral development of the child. For example, maternal anxiety, but not antenatal depression is linked to a difficult child temperament at the age of 4–6 months [19], an increase in behavioral and emotional problems at the age of 4 [20] and more internalizing behavior at the age of 8 [21]. Moreover, antenatal depression is associated with delayed development in 18-month-olds [22], increased externalizing behaviors and a slight decrease in IQ in 8-year-old children [21], and violent behavior during adolescence [23]. On the long-term prenatal exposure to maternal depression is associated with a higher chance of developing depression during adolescence [24, 25] and adulthood [26], or risk of developing other psychopathologies [27]. Maternal anxiety as well as maternal depression during pregnancy is correlated with child attention problems at the age of 3 and 4 [28]. Moreover, an increase in reporting symptoms of antenatal depression and anxiety positively correlated with an increase in internalizing behaviors in 4-year-olds [29]. So anxiety and depression appear to have similar but, at the same time, different effects on offspring development; however, it is difficult to discern between maternal anxiety and depression, due to common comorbidity between these mental health conditions [30].

Overall, maternal vulnerability, such as depression and anxiety, during pregnancy can negatively influence the unborn child on both physiological and behavioral levels. However, it remains difficult to discern the direct effects of antenatal depression (an aversive postnatal environment due to a depressed mother), and genetic predisposition to vulnerability on fetal and infant development. In addition, an increasing percentage of women suffering from depression and/or anxiety are treated with antidepressants, which on itself might have tremendous effects on the developing child.

2. Maternal SSRI treatment and offspring development

Pharmacological treatment of antenatal depression and/or anxiety is sometimes unavoidable. The treatment with antidepressants may relieve the symptoms of the depression of the mother and could help in reducing the impact on the unborn child. Nowadays, a considerable number of women are treated with antidepressants during pregnancy. In Europe, this concerns 2–3% of the pregnant women [16, 31], while in the U.S., the occurrence is as high as up to 13% [32, 33]. The most prescribed antidepressants are selective serotonin reuptake inhibitors (SSRIs), because of their good efficacy, few side effects, and therapeutic safety [34]. These drugs work by blocking the serotonin transporter and hereby preventing the reabsorption of the neurotransmitter serotonin into the presynaptic nerve cell. Subsequently, extracellular serotonin levels in the synaptic cleft are increased and more serotonin is available to bind the postsynaptic receptors. Although, SSRIs are considered safe for antenatal use [35], it has been reported that the use of SSRIs during pregnancy may negatively influence the development of the unborn child. SSRIs can cross the placenta and are found in the amniotic fluid [36, 37], affecting therefore not only the mother but also the developing child. This is of extra concern as serotonin plays a key role in embryonal development. During the development of the fetal brain, serotonin acts as a neurotrophic factor, regulating cell division, differentiation, migration, growth cone elongation, dendritic pruning, myelination, and synaptogenesis [38]. In fact, serotonin receptors and serotonergic metabolic enzymes are expressed before serotonin-producing neurons are present in the brain [39]. Thus, changes in the serotonin levels during neurodevelopment, for instance, by the administration of SSRIs during pregnancy, potentially affect a number of processes in the offspring.

Indeed, literature shows a number of side effects in the offspring due to prenatal SSRI exposure. First of all, SSRI exposure during pregnancy has been associated with attenuated basal cortisol levels in neonates [40, 41], and differential cortisol levels in 3-month-old infants in response to a stressor [42]. Also, the neonatal heart rate response to an acute noxious event is attenuated [43]. Furthermore, several behavioral changes have been reported, such as increased internalizing behaviors, such as depression, anxiety, and social withdrawal during childhood [44, 45], increased externalizing behaviors in 4-year-old children [46], and disrupted sleep patterns in newborn [47]. In addition, SSRIs reduce utero-placental blood flow, a mechanism thought to be involved with hypertension in preeclampsia and gestational diabetes [48, 49].

Recently, there has been much interest in the link between antenatal SSRI treatment and the development of autism spectrum disorders (ASDs) in the child. ASD is a neurodevelopmental condition characterized by difficulties in social communication and unusually restricted, repetitive behavior and interests. The available literature shows an association between the prenatal use of SSRIs and the increased risk of ASDs in the child [50–54]. It is theorized that this is facilitated by an increase in serotonergic activity during brain development [55]. Several studies found abnormal placental histology to be associated with autism diagnosis [56, 57]. Moreover, autistic patients have elevated blood platelet serotonin levels [58, 59]. Taken together, these results imply the serotonergic influences on maternal-fetal interaction, although the exact mechanisms remain elusive.

A possible route for passing adverse intra-uterine effects to the fetus is via epigenetic regulation. For example, increased maternal depressive mood during pregnancy is associated with reduced methylation of the promotor of the gene coding the serotonin transporter (SERT) in both mothers and newborns [60]. These results suggest increased SERT mRNA levels and subsequently modified serotonin levels, contributing to increased vulnerability later in life [61]. St-Pierre and colleagues therefore conclude that all parameters that can alter serotonin homeostasis during early development could lead to structural and functional changes in fetal development and brain circuits [62], which could subsequently result in a predisposition to psychopathology in adulthood.

Thus, several studies have shown an increased risk for developing the child both during antenatal depression and after prenatal SSRI exposure. However, it is difficult to discern between the effects of the SSRIs and the effects of the depression itself, as healthy mothers do not administer antidepressants. For example, meta-analyses show that the risk found for ASD in the offspring after prenatal SSRI exposure is decreased after correcting for maternal mental illness [63]. Thus, the effects of SSRIs mentioned could be solely due to the administration of the SSRIs, or alternatively, the SSRIs are only partially effective and therefore do not eliminate all the adverse effects of the depression, thereby adding up to the adverse effects of antenatal depression [4].

3. Preclinical studies: perinatal SSRI exposure

In humans, it is difficult, if not impossible, to discern the effects of the SSRI and the depression itself on fetal development. It is not ethical to study the effects of SSRIs in healthy pregnant women. In addition, it is impossible to study gene expression and epigenetic changes in the fetal brain as a result of prenatal SSRI exposure. Due to these limitations of human research, researchers often use animal models, specifically rodents, to get a more profound insight into the mechanisms underlying the observations seen in human studies.

It should be noted that the timing of brain development is different in humans compared to rodents. A rodent brain at postnatal day 7–10 is considered to be the rough equivalent of a newborn human infant [64]. Thus, to mimic SSRI exposure during the entire pregnancy in humans, rodents should be exposed both pre- and postnatally. In addition, it is known that SSRIs are also found in breast milk [65], again underlining the need to research both the effects of pre- and postnatal SSRI exposure. For exposure to SSRIs around these time points, we will use the term perinatal SSRI exposure; when timing of the SSRI exposure is of particular importance, we will distinguish between pre- and postnatal exposure to SSRIs.

3.1 Social behavior

As serotonin is a key regulator of social responses and prenatal SSRI exposure is being linked to ASDs, which are characterized by impaired social behavior [54], this behavioral parameter is often addressed in researching the effects of prenatal SSRI exposure in animals.

Social play at juvenile age is an essential behavior in rodents for the development of the necessary social, cognitive, emotional, and physical skills [66]. SSRIs are well described in literature as reducing social play behavior in young rats when prenatally [67] or postnatally [68–71] administered. These effects of SSRIs seem sex-mediated, as males are more affected than females [70], or females are not even affected at all [71]. This is interesting because this is analogous to the situation, where men are 3–4 times more likely to get diagnosed with ASDs compared to women [72]. In spite of that, not all studies found similar results. In a recent study [73], social play behavior was unaltered after prenatal SSRI exposure. However, in the latter study, social play was assessed with a familiar play partner (littermate), while other studies use a novel conspecific.

Findings on the effects of prenatal SSRI exposure on social behavior at adult age are more conflicting. Olivier and colleagues [67] found reduced social exploration in adult male rats after prenatal SSRI exposure. While another study found that 4 days of postnatal treatment with SSRIs led to increased sniffing, contact with, and total social interaction with a novel conspecific in males [74]. On top of that, other studies found no effect of prenatal SSRI exposure on social exploration in both males and females [75, 76]. In general, studies on the exposure of SSRIs during early development on adult social interaction are unconvincing. Studies on social motivation on the other hand, measured as the preference of a rodent to spend time with a novel conspecific over interaction with an object, appear to be more in line. Decreased social motivation is found in both males and females, when postnatally exposed to SSRIs [69–71, 77]. On the other hand, prenatal exposure to SSRIs led to an increase in motivation to interact with a conspecific in mice [75]. Thus, while literature on the effects of perinatal SSRI exposure on social behavior during adult is still limited, both timing of the exposure and sex are important factors in the subsequent social development.

Another form of social interaction under the influence of the neurotransmitter serotonin is aggression [78]. Indeed, during both childhood and adulthood, SSRIs are successfully used to reduce aggressive and violent behavior in certain mental disorders

[79, 80]. Perinatal exposure to SSRIs, on the other hand, leads to increased externalizing behavior, such as aggression, in children [46]. In rodents, the effects of perinatal SSRI exposure on aggressive behavior are conflicting. Several studies show an increase in male, but not female aggressive behavior [73, 75, 76, 81], while other studies show reduced aggressive behavior in male rodents perinatally exposed to SSRIs [82, 83].

Serotonin is known to be involved in the regulation of maternal care [84]. Thus, perinatal SSRI exposure can be expected to alter maternal caregiving behavior of both the SSRI-treated mother and her female offspring, when they are mothers later in life. Typical maternal behaviors include nest building, gathering the young into the nest, maternal licking, and nursing the pups. Studies on the effect of direct SSRI exposure found an increase in these behaviors [85, 86], or no effect at all [87]. So far, only one study has been performed on the effects of prenatal exposure on maternal care later in life, and interestingly here, they found a reduction in maternal caregiving behaviors [75]. This suggests that direct changes in serotonin levels, such as an increase in extracellular serotonin levels during SSRI treatment and changes in serotonin levels during development differentially alter the quality of maternal care.

Another role for serotonin is its signaling in sexual development, on both the brain and at a behavioral level [88]. In addition, chronic SSRI treatment may result in sexual dysfunction [89]. Not much is known on the effect of perinatal SSRI exposure on the sexual behavior of these children later in life; however, several studies have been performed in rodents. The effect of perinatal SSRI exposure depends on the timing of treatment. When postnatally administered, male sexual behavior later in life is reduced [70, 90–93]. In contrast when the SSRI is prenatally, or both prenatally and postnatally, administered, there is no effect on sexual behavior of male rodents [94, 95]. Interestingly, there appears to be an opposite effect in female offspring, where postnatal SSRI exposure leads to an increase in sexual behaviors [75, 96]. Thus, apart from the effect of timing, sex of the offspring also differentially alters the effect of perinatal SSRI exposure on reproductive behavior.

3.2 Affective behavior

It has long been established that serotonin is involved in affective disorders [97]. Affective disorders, also called mood disorders, include psychiatric disorders such as major depressive disorder and anxiety disorders.

A large body of preclinical research has shown the relationship between perinatal SSRI exposure and anxiety. Although there are some studies finding no effects, several studies did find an increase in anxiety-like behavior and/or less explorative behavior in an open field test, when rodents are perinatally exposed to SSRIs [67, 83, 98–104]. An increase in anxiety-like behavior in the elevated plus maze and the novelty-suppressed feeding test are also found [67, 98, 99, 105]. Nevertheless, there are also studies that did not find effects at all [87, 91, 106–111], and two studies even found a decrease in behaviors related to anxiety [92, 112]. Even though results differ among studies, these differences are not clearly linked to sex of the offspring or timing of the SSRI exposure. So even though there appears to be a clear link between perinatal SSRI exposure and anxiety later in life, to get a more profound insight into the mechanisms behind this and the role of timing and sex, more researches have to be done.

It is difficult to determine if a rodent is depressed, moreover, to determine if it is even possible for rodents to experience depression. However, rodents can show behavior characteristics of the behaviors, and humans show during episodes of major depression. Such behaviors encompass despair and anhedonia [113]. To measure behavioral despair in rodents, the forced swim test is usually performed [114]. In this test, the animal is placed in an unescapable container filled with water, forcing the rodent to swim. After making efforts to escape the animal may eventually stop his efforts and become immobile. The amount of time spent immobile is used as a measure of helplessness and behavioral despair. As reviewed [115], many, but not all, studies performing the forced swim test after perinatal SSRI exposure found an increase in immobility [83, 99, 100, 105, 106, 109, 110, 116–121]. Three studies did not find an effect [67, 87, 111], and three studies even found a decrease in immobility [103, 112, 122]. The reviewers propose that these differences may be due to strain effects, some strains could be more susceptible to early life SSRI exposure, while others are resistant. In addition, they point out that the effect of perinatal SSRI exposure is greater, when the animals are exposed during early postnatal period rather than the prenatal period.

Anhedonia is another behavior often assessed as a measure for depression. Anhedonia is the inability or lack of motivation to experience pleasure from rewarding activities and is measured in rodents with the sucrose preference test [123]. In this test, two drinking bottles are placed in the rodent's home cage. One is filled with water and the other with a sucrose solution. Preference for the sucrose solution is considered as the typical hedonic behavior, and lack of bias toward the sucrose water is characterized as a sign of anhedonia. It appears that only postnatal SSRI exposure increases anhedonia later in life [124], as opposed to prenatal exposure [67, 125]. This once more emphasizes that the moment of exposure is an important factor in assessing the effects of perinatal SSRI exposure.

Thus, not only sex of the offspring, but also the timing of the SSRI exposure appears to play an important role in behavioral development. However, all aforementioned studies are performed in offspring from healthy mothers. In practice, pregnant women are usually treated with SSRIs when they are suffering from anxiety and/or depression. It is likely that both maternal factors and the treatment with SSRIs affect serotonin functioning in the embryo and infant. The interplay of these two factors might shape the development of the fetus in a different way than antenatal depression or prenatal SSRI exposure on its own. Thus, to make a more valid translational step to the human situation, animal models of maternal vulnerability have to be used.

4. Preclinical studies: maternal vulnerability and perinatal SSRI exposure

To induce maternal vulnerability in healthy rodents, researchers often use the early life stress model (ELS). Maternal separation is one of the manipulations often used to create ELS; in this procedure, the offspring is taken away from the mother for few hours during the day, and this happens daily during a period of few early postnatal weeks. This procedure leads to a long-term and intergenerational increase in anxiety and depressive-like behaviors [126–131]. Female offspring exposed to ELS and showing an increase in anxiety and depressive-live behaviors can be used as a model of maternal vulnerability later in life. Little is known about the interaction of such maternal vulnerability and treatment with SSRIs during pregnancy.

4.1 Social behavior

So far, only two studies have been looking into the combined effects of maternal vulnerability and perinatal SSRI exposure on social play behavior and social interaction of the offspring later in life. In 2017, Gemmel and colleagues [73] showed that the reduction in social play behavior in juveniles due to maternal vulnerability is prevented by perinatal SSRI treatment regardless of the sex of the offspring. This suggests a rescuing effect of SSRIs on social behavior in offspring of stressed mothers. However, social aggressive play was increased in adolescent offspring exposed to perinatal fluoxetine and maternal vulnerability in both sexes. In addition, time grooming a novel conspecific was decreased in males only. In a later study, Gemmel and colleagues [132] did not find such an interaction effect on social behavior in adult offspring. Even though, maternal vulnerability itself decreased social investigation in adult males while perinatal SSRI exposure increased social investigation in adult females and increased social play in adult males. Thus, normalization, by SSRIs, of altered social play and social interaction, due to maternal vulnerability might only be short-lived as it does not persist into adulthood. With regard to aggression, however, long-term protective effects of SSRIs are found [81]. In this study, aggressive behavior was decreased as a result of maternal vulnerability, which was normalized when perinatal SSRI exposure was included in the treatment.

One study has looked into the combined effect of SSRI exposure and maternal vulnerability on offspring sexual development [133]. Perinatal SSRI exposure reduced sexual behavior in male offspring, while interestingly maternal vulnerability alone or the combination of maternal vulnerability and perinatal SSRI exposure did not have any effect on the development of sexual behavior.

So, even though SSRI treatment of vulnerable mothers appears to have protective effects on offspring social development, these findings are not consistent over all types of behavior and differ with the moment of assessment of the offspring.

4.2 Affective behavior

Affective behaviors of the offspring such as anxiety and depression-like behaviors have also been studied after the offspring was exposed to a combination of maternal vulnerability and perinatal SSRI exposure. One study [134] shows that the increase in anxiety due to maternal vulnerability can be reversed by the postnatal administration of SSRIs. When prenatally administered, such a rescuing effect is not found [87]; however, the effect of maternal vulnerability was limited and was only found in males in this study. Two studies assessed depressive-like behavior after perinatal exposure to both maternal vulnerability and SSRIs. Both studies found that SSRIs normalize the increase in immobility in the forced swim test due to maternal vulnerability [87, 135]. Thus so far, the effect maternal vulnerability has on anxiety and depressive-like symptoms in the offspring later in life appear to be reversed by SSRIs.

5. Conclusion

Thus, children from mothers who suffer from anxiety or major depression during their pregnancy are at risk of developing several psychopathologies later in life. Moreover, treatment with SSRIs during pregnancy can also lead to long-term consequences for the children. However, it is difficult to determine if these effects are due to the SSRI treatment, maternal vulnerability, or a combination of both. Preclinical research in rodents shows that perinatal SSRI exposure on itself leads to alterations in social behavior later in life. Specifically, social play in juveniles, sexual behavior, maternal care in females, and aggression in males are influenced. Affective behaviors are also influenced, and both anxiety and depressive-like behaviors are increased due to perinatal SSRI exposure. Both the moments of SSRI exposure, pre- or postnatal, and sex of the offspring appear to be important factors in the development of social and affective behaviors after perinatal SSRI treatment.

Recently, researchers have started to look into the combined effects of maternal vulnerability and perinatal SSRI exposure in preclinical studies to make a more valid translational step to the human situation. Even though only a few studies have been done so far, it seems that, at least some, developmental alterations on offspring behavior due to maternal vulnerability can be normalized by perinatal SSRI exposure. These are interesting and promising results and further investigation into the risks and benefits of SSRI use during pregnancy in appropriate animal models are necessary to help depressed women in their decision to use SSRIs during pregnancy.

Conflict of interest

The authors declare that there is no conflict of interest.

Author details

Laura Staal and Jocelien DA Olivier*
Neurobiology, Groningen Institute for Evolutionary Life Sciences, Groningen, The Netherlands

*Address all correspondence to: j.d.a.olivier@rug.nl

References

[1] Ryan D, Milis L, Misri N. Depression during pregnancy. Canadian Family Physician. 2005;**51**:1087-1093

[2] Melville JL, Gavin A, Guo Y, Fan M, Katon WJ. Depressive disorders during pregnancy: Prevalence and risk factors in a large urban sample. Obstetrics and Gynecology. 2010;**116**(5):1064-1070

[3] Kim DR, Snell JL, Ewing GC, O'Reardon J. Neuromodulation and antenatal depression: A review. Neuropsychiatric Disease and Treatment. 2015;**11**:975-982

[4] Olivier JDA, Åkerud H, Sundström I. Antenatal depression and antidepressants during pregnancy: Unraveling the complex interactions for the offspring. European Journal of Pharmacology. 2015;**753**:257-262

[5] Field T, Diego M, Hernandez-reif M. Prenatal depression effects on the fetus and newborn: A review. Infant Behavior & Development. 2006;**29**:445-455

[6] Gitau R, Cameron A, Fisk NM, Glover V. Fetal exposure to maternal cortisol. Lancet. 1998;**352**:707-708

[7] Kaplan LA, Evans L, Monk C. Effects of mothers' prenatal psychiatric status and postnatal caregiving on infant biobehavioral regulation: Can prenatal programming be modified? Early Human Development. 2008;**84**(4):249-256

[8] Ellman LM, Schetter CD, Hobel CJ, Chicz-DeMet A, Glynn LM, Sandman CA. Timing of fetal exposure to stress hormones: Effects on newborn physical and neuromuscular maturation. Developmental Psychobiology. 2008;**50**(3):232-241

[9] Davis EP, Glynn LM, Waffarn F, Sandman CA. Prenatal maternal stress programs infant stress regulation. Journal of Child Psychology and Psychiatry. 2011;**52**(2):119-129

[10] Davis EP, Snidman N, Wadhwa PD, Glynn LM, Schetter CD, Sandman CA. Prenatal maternal anxiety and depression predict negative behavioral reactivity in infancy. Infancy. 2004;**6**(3):319-331

[11] Davis EP, Glynn LM, Schetter CD, Hobel C, Chicz-Demet A, Sandman CA. Prenatal exposure to maternal depression and cortisol influences infant temperament. Journal of the American Academy of Child and Adolescent Psychiatry. 2007;**46**(6):737-746

[12] Huizink AC, Robles de Medina PG, EJH M, GHA V, Buitelaar JK. Stress during pregnancy is associatedwith developmental outcome in infancy. Journal of Child Psychology and Psychiatry. 2003;**44**(6):810-818

[13] Mennes M, Stiers P, Lagae L, Van den Bergh B. Long-term cognitive sequelae of antenatal maternal anxiety: Involvement of the orbitofrontal cortex. Neuroscience and Biobehavioral Reviews. 2006;**30**:1078-1086

[14] Field T, Diego M, Hernandez-Reif M, Figueiredo B, Schanberg S, Kuhn C. Sleep disturbances in depressed pregnant women and their newborns. Infant Behavior & Development. 2007;**30**:127-133

[15] O'Connor TG, Caprariello P, Blackmore ER, Gregory AM, Glover V, Fleming P. Prenatal mood disturbance predicts sleep problems in infancy and toddlerhood. Early Human Development. 2007;**83**(7):451-458

[16] El Marroun H, Jaddoe VWV, Hudziak JJ, Roza SJ, Steegers EAP, Hofman A, et al. Maternal use of selective serotonin reuptake inhibitors, fetal growth, and risk of adverse

birth outcomes. Archives of General Psychiatry. 2012;**69**(7):706-714

[17] Henrichs J, Schenk JJ, Roza SJ, van den Berg MP, Schmidt HG, Steegers EAP, et al. Maternal psychological distress and fetal growth trajectories: The generation R study. Psychological Medicine. 2010;**40**:633-643

[18] Fan F, Zou Y, Tian H, Zhang Y, Zhang J, Ma X, et al. Effects of maternal anxiety and depression during pregnancy in Chinese women on children's heart rate and blood pressure response to stress. Journal of Human Hypertension. 2016;**30**:171-176

[19] Austin MP, Hadzi-Pavlovic D, Leader L, Saint K, Parker G. Maternal trait anxiety, depression and life event stress in pregnancy: Relationships with infant temperament. Early Human Development. 2005;**81**:183-190

[20] O'Connor TG, Heron J, Glover V. Antenatal anxiety predicts child behavioral/emotional problems independently of postnatal depression. Journal of the American Academy of Child and Adolescent Psychiatry. 2002;**41**(12):1470-1477

[21] Barker ED, Jaffee SR, Uher R, Maughan B. The contribution of prenatal and postnatal maternal anxiety and depression to child maladjustment. Depression and Anxiety. 2011;**28**(8):696-702

[22] Deave T, Heron J, Evans J, Emond A. The impact of maternal depression in pregnancy on early child development. BJOG : An International Journal of Obstetrics and Gynaecology. 2008;**115**:1043-1051

[23] Hay DF, Pawlby S, Waters CS, Perra O, Sharp D. Mothers' antenatal depression and their children's antisocial outcomes. Child Development. 2010;**81**(1):149-165

[24] Plant DT, Pariante CM, Sharp D, Pawlby S. Maternal depression during pregnancy and offspring depression in adulthood: Role of child maltreatment. The British Journal of Psychiatry. 2015;**207**:213-220

[25] Pawlby S, Hay DF, Waters CS, Sharp D, O'Keane V. Antenatal depression predicts depression in adolescent offspring: Prospective longitudinal community-based study. Journal of Affective Disorders. 2009;**113**(3):236-243

[26] Pearson RM, Evans J, Kounali D, Lewis G, Heron J, Ramchandani PG, et al. Maternal depression during pregnancy and the postnatal period risks and possible mechanisms for offspring depression at age 18 years. JAMA Psychiatry. 2013;**70**(12):1312-1319

[27] Pawlby S, Hay D, Sharp D, Waters CS, Pariante CM. Antenatal depression and offspring psychopathology: The influence of childhood maltreatment. The British Journal of Psychiatry. 2011;**199**:106-112

[28] Van Batenburg-Eddes T, Brion MJ, Henrichs J, Jaddoe VWV, Hofman A, Verhulst FC, et al. Parental depressive and anxiety symptoms during pregnancy and attention problems in children: A cross-cohort consistency study. Journal of Child Psychology and Psychiatry. 2012;**54**(5):591-600

[29] Misri S, Reebye P, Kendrick K, Carter D, Ryan D, Grunau RE, et al. Internalizing behaviors in 4-year-old children exposed in utero to psychotropic medications. The American Journal of Psychiatry. 2006;**163**:1026-1032

[30] Glover V. Maternal depression, anxiety and stress during pregnancy and child outcome; what needs to be done. Best Practice & Research. Clinical Obstetrics & Gynaecology. 2014;**28**(1):25-35

[31] Kieler H, Artama M, Engeland A, Ericsson Ö, Furu K, Gissler M, et al. Selective serotonin reuptake inhibitors during pregnancy and risk of persistent pulmonary hypertension in the newborn: Population based cohort study from the five Nordic countries. BMJ. 2012;**344**:1-9

[32] Cooper WO, Willy ME, Pont SJ, Ray WA. Increasing use of antidepressants in pregnancy. American Journal of Obstetrics and Gynecology. 2007;**196**:1-5

[33] Hayes RM, Wu DP, Shelton RC, Cooper O, Dupont WD, Mitchel E, et al. Maternal antidepressant use and adverse outcomes: A cohort study of 228,876 pregnancies. American Journal of Obstetrics and Gynecology. 2012;**207**(1):49

[34] Barbey JT, Roose SP. SSRI safety in overdose. The Journal of Clinical Psychiatry. 1998;**59**:42-48

[35] Gentile S. The safety of newer antidepressantsin pregnancy and breastfeeding. Drug Safety. 2005;**28**(2):137-152

[36] Hostetter A, Stowe ZN, Strader JR, McLaughlin E, Llewellyn A. Dose of selective serotonin uptake inhibitors across pregnancy: Clinical implications. Depression and Anxiety. 2000;**11**(2):51-57

[37] Loughhead AM, Fisher AD, Newport DJ, Ritchie JC, Owens MJ, CL DV, et al. Antidepressants in amniotic fluid: Another route of fetal exposure. The American Journal of Psychiatry. 2006;**163**(1):145-147

[38] Gaspar P, Cases O, Maroteaux L. The developmental role of serotonin: News from mouse molecular genetics. Nature Reviews. Neuroscience. 2003;**4**(12):1002-1012

[39] Bonnin A, Goeden N, Chen K, Wilson ML, King J, Shih JC, et al. A transient placental source of serotonin for the fetal forebrain. Nature. 2011;**472**(7343):347-350

[40] Brennan PA, Pargas R, Walker EF, Green P, Jeffrey Newport D, Stowe Z. Maternal depression and infant cortisol: Influences of timing, comorbidity and treatment. The Journal of Child Psychology and Psychiatry and Allied Disciplines. 2008;**49**(10):1099-1107

[41] Pawluski JL, Brain UM, Underhill CM, Hammond GL, Oberlander TF. Prenatal SSRI exposure alters neonatal corticosteroid binding globulin, infant cortisol levels, and emerging HPA function. Psychoneuroendocrinology. 2012;**37**(7):1019-1028

[42] Oberlander TF, Grunau R, Mayes L, Riggs W, Rurak D, Papsdorf M, et al. Hypothalamic-pituitary-adrenal (HPA) axis function in 3-month old infants with prenatal selective serotonin reuptake inhibitor (SSRI) antidepressant exposure. Early Human Development. 2008;**84**(10):689-697

[43] Oberlander TF, Eckstein Grunau R, Fitzgerald C, Ellwood A-L, Misri S, Rurak D, et al. Prolonged prenatal psychotropic medication exposure alters neonatal acute pain response. Pediatric Research. 2002;**51**(4):443-453

[44] Hanley GE, Brain U, Oberlander TF. Prenatal exposure to serotonin reuptake inhibitor antidepressants and childhood behavior. Pediatric Research. 2015;**78**:174-180

[45] Oberlander TF, Papsdorf M, Brain UM, Misri S, Ross C, Grunau RE. Prenatal effects of selective serotonin reuptake inhibitor antidepressants, serotonin transporter promoter genotype. Archives of Pediatrics & Adolescent Medicine. 2010;**164**(5):444-451

[46] Oberlander TF, Reebye P, Misri S, Papsdorf M, Kim J, Grunau RE.

Externalizing and attentional behaviors in children of depressed mothers treated with a selective serotonin reuptake inhibitor antidepressant during pregnancy. Archives of Pediatrics & Adolescent Medicine. 2007;**161**:22-29

[47] Zeskind PS, Stephens LE. Maternal selective serotonin reuptake inhibitor use during pregnancy and newborn neurobehavior. Pediatrics. 2004;**113**(2):368-375

[48] Bolte AC, Van Geijn HP, Dekker GA. Pathophysiology of preeclampsia and the role of serotonin. European Journal of Obstetrics, Gynecology, and Reproductive Biology. 2001;**95**(1):12-21

[49] Li Y, Hadden C, Singh P, Mercado CP, Murphy P, Dajani NK, et al. GDM-associated insulin deficiency hinders the dissociation of SERT from ERp44 and down-regulates placental 5-HT uptake. Proceedings of the National Academy of Sciences of the United States of America. 2014;**111**(52):E5697-E5705

[50] Andalib S, Emamhadi MR, Yousefzadeh-Chabok S, Shakouri SK, Høilund-Carlsen PF, Vafaee MS, et al. Maternal SSRI exposure increases the risk of autistic offspring: A meta-analysis and systematic review. European Psychiatry. 2017;**45**:161-166. DOI: 10.1016/j.eurpsy.2017.06.001

[51] Brown HK, Hussain-Shamsy N, Lunsky Y, Dennis CLE, Vigod SN. The association between antenatal exposure to selective serotonin reuptake inhibitors and autism: A systematic review and meta-analysis. The Journal of Clinical Psychiatry. 2017;**78**:e48-e58

[52] Kaplan YC, Keskin-Arslan E, Acar S, Sozmen K. Prenatal selective serotonin reuptake inhibitor use and the risk of autism spectrum disorder in children: A systematic review and meta-analysis. Reproductive Toxicology. 2016;**66**:31-43

[53] Kobayashi T, Matsuyama T, Takeuchi M, Ito S. Autism spectrum disorder and prenatal exposure to selective serotonin reuptake inhibitors: A systematic review and meta-analysis. Reproductive Toxicology. 2016;**65**: 170-178. DOI: 10.1016/j.reprotox.2016.07.016

[54] Gentile S. Prenatal antidepressant exposure and the risk of autism spectrum disorders in children. Are we looking at the fall of gods? Journal of Affective Disorders. 2015;**182**:132-137

[55] Whitaker-Azmitia PM. Behavioral and cellular consequences of increasing serotonergic activity during brain development: A role in autism? International Journal of Developmental Neuroscience. 2005;**23**(1):75-83

[56] Anderson GM, Gutknecht L, Cohen DJ, Brailly-Tabard S, Cohen JHM, Ferrari P, et al. Serotonin transporter promoter variants in autism: Functional effects and relationship to platelet hyperserotonemia. Molecular Psychiatry. 2002;**7**(8):831-836

[57] Walker CK, Anderson KW, Milano KM, Ye S, Tancredi DJ, Pessah IN, et al. Trophoblast inclusions are significantly increased in the placentas of childeren in families at risk for autism. Biological Psychiatry. 2013;**74**(3):204-211

[58] McBride PA, Anderson GM, Hertzig ME, Snow ME, Thompson SM, Khait VD, et al. Effects of diagnosis, race, and puberty on platelet serotonin levels in autism and mental retardation. Journal of the American Academy of Child and Adolescent Psychiatry. 1998;**37**(7):767-776

[59] Bijl N, Thys C, Wittevrongel C, De La Marche W, Devriendt K, Peeters H, et al. Platelet studies in autism spectrum disorder patients and first-degree relatives. Molecular Autism. 2015;**6**(1):1-10

[60] Devlin AM, Brain U, Austin J, Oberlander TF. Prenatal exposure to

maternal depressed mood and the MTHFR C677T variant affect SLC6A4 methylation in infants at birth. PLoS One. 2010;**5**(8):2-9

[61] Philibert R, Madan A, Andersen A, Cadoret R, Packer H, Sandhu H. Serotonin transporter mRNA levels are associated with the methylation of an upstream CpG island. American Journal of Medical Genetics. 2007;**144B**:101-105

[62] St-Pierre J, Laurent L, King S, Vaillancourt C. Effects of prenatal maternal stress on serotonin and fetal development. Placenta. 2016;**48**:S66-S71

[63] Andrade C. Antidepressant exposure during pregnancy and risk of autism in the offspring, 1: Meta-review of meta-analyses. The Journal of Clinical Psychiatry. 2017;**78**(8):e48-e58

[64] Semple B, Blomgren K, Gimlin K, Ferriero D, Noble-Haeusslein L. Brain development in rodents and humans: Identifying benchmarks of maturation and vulnerability to injury across species. Progress in Neurobiology. 2013:1-16

[65] Heikkinen T, Ekblad U, Palo P, Laine K. Pharmacokinetics of fluoxetine and norfluoxetine in pregnancy and lactation. Clinical Pharmacology and Therapeutics. 2003;**73**(4):330-337

[66] Vanderschuren LJ, Trezza V. What the laboratory rat has taught us about social play behavior: Role in behavioral development and neural mechanisms. Current Topics in Behavioral Neurosciences. 2014;**16**:189-212

[67] Olivier JDA, Vallès A, Van Heesch F, Afrasiab-Middelman A, Roelofs JJPM, Jonkers M, et al. Fluoxetine administration to pregnant rats increases anxiety-related behavior in the offspring. Psychopharmacology. 2011;**217**(3):419-432

[68] Homberg JR, Schiepers OJG, Schoffelmeer ANM, Cuppen E, Vanderschuren LJMJ. Acute and constitutive increases in central serotonin levels reduce social play behaviour in peri-adolescent rats. Psychopharmacology. 2007;**195**(2):175-182

[69] Khatri N, Simpson KL, Lin RCS, Paul IA. Lasting neurobehavioral abnormalities in rats after neonatal activation of serotonin 1A and 1B receptors: Possible mechanisms for serotonin dysfunction in autistic spectrum disorders. Psychopharmacologia. 2014;**231**(6):1191-1200

[70] Rodriguez-Porcel F, Green D, Khatri N, Swilley Harris S, May WL, Lin RCS, et al. Neonatal exposure of rats to antidepressants affects behavioral reactions to novelty and social interactions in a manner analogous to autistic spectrum disorders. The Anatomical Record. 2011;**294**(10):1726-1735

[71] Simpson KL, Weaver KJ, de Villers-Sidani E, Lu JY-F, Cai Z, Pang Y, et al. Perinatal antidepressant exposure alters cortical network function in rodents. PNAS. 2011;**108**(45):18465-18470

[72] Christensen DL, Bilder DA, Zahorodny W, Pettygrove S, Durkin MS, Fitzgerald RT, et al. Prevalence and characteristics of autism spectrum disorder among 4-year-old children in the autism and developmental disabilities monitoring network. Journal of Developmental and Behavioral Pediatrics. 2016;**37**:1-8

[73] Gemmel M, Hazlett M, Bögi E, De Lacalle S, Hill LA, Kokras N, et al. Perinatal fluoxetine effects on social play, the HPA system, and hippocampal plasticity in pre-adolescent male and female rats: Interactions with pre-gestational maternal stress. Psychoneuroendocrinology. 2017;**84**:159-171

[74] Ko MC, Lee LJH, Li Y, Lee LJ. Long-term consequences of neonatal fluoxetine exposure in adult rats. Developmental Neurobiology. 2014;**74**(10):1038-1051

[75] Svirsky N, Levy S, Avitsur R. Prenatal exposure to selective serotonin reuptake inhibitors (SSRI) increases aggression and modulates maternal behavior in offspring mice. Developmental Psychobiology. 2016;**58**(1):71-82

[76] Kiryanova V, Dyck RH. Increased aggression, improved spatial memory, and reduced anxiety-like behaviour in adult male mice exposed to fluoxetine early in life. Developmental Neuroscience. 2014;**36**(5):396-408

[77] Zimmerberg B, Germeyan SC. Effects of neonatal fluoxetine exposure on behavior across development in rats selectively bred for an infantile affective trait. Developmental Psychobiology. 2015;**57**(2):141-152

[78] Duke AA, Bègue L, Bell R, Eisenlohr-moul T. Revisiting the serotonin-aggression relation in humans: A meta-analysis. Psychological Bulletin. 2013;**139**(5):1148-1172

[79] Blader JC. Pharmacotherapy and postdischarge outcomes of child inpatients admitted for aggressive behavior. Journal of Clinical Psychopharmacology. 2006;**26**(4):419-425

[80] Bond AJ. Antidepressant treatments and human aggression. European Journal of Pharmacology. 2005;**526**(1-3):218-225

[81] Kiryanova V, Meunier SJ, Vecchiarelli HA, Hill MN, Dyck RH. Effects of maternal stress and perinatal fluoxetine exposure on behavioral outcomes of adult male offspring. Neuroscience. 2016;**320**:281-296

[82] Manhaes De Castro R, Barreto Medeiros JM, Mendes Da Silva C, Ferreira LMP, Guedes RCA, Cabrai Filho JE, et al. Reduction of intraspecific aggression in adult rats by neonatal treatment with a selective serotonin reuptake inhibitor. Brazilian Journal of Medical and Biological Research. 2001;**34**(1):121-124

[83] Lisboa SFS, Oliveira PE, Costa LC, Venâncio EJ, Moreira EG. Behavioral evaluation of male and female mice pups exposed to fluoxetine during pregnancy and lactation. Pharmacology. 2007;**80**(1):49-56

[84] Zoratto F, Fiore M, Ali SF, Laviola G, Macrì S. Neonatal tryptophan depletion and corticosterone supplementation modify emotional responses in adult male mice. Psychoneuroendocrinology. 2013;**38**(1):24-39

[85] Johns JM, Joyner PW, McMurray MS, Elliot DL, Hofler VE, Middleton CL, et al. The effects of dopaminergic/serotonergic reuptake inhibition on maternal behavior, maternal aggression, and oxytocin in the rat. Pharmacology, Biochemistry, and Behavior. 2005;**81**(4):769-785

[86] Pawluski JL, Charlier TD, Fillet M, Houbart V, Crispin HT, Steinbusch HW, et al. Chronic fluoxetine treatment and maternal adversity differentially alter neurobehavioral outcomes in the rat dam. Behavioural Brain Research. 2012;**228**(1):159-168

[87] Rayen I, van den Hove DL, Prickaerts J, Steinbusch HW, Pawluski JL. Fluoxetine during development reverses the effects of prenatal stress on depressive-like behavior and hippocampal neurogenesis in adolescence. PLoS One. 2011;**6**(9):e24003

[88] Dohler KD, Jarzab B, Sickmoller PM, Kokocinska D, Kaminski M, Gubala E,

et al. Influence of neurotransmitters on sexual differentiation of brain structure and function. Experimental and Clinical Endocrinology. 1991;**98**:99-109

[89] Balon R. SSRI-associated sexual dysfunction. The American Journal of Psychiatry. 2006;**163**(9): 1504-1509

[90] Gouvea TS, Morimoto HK, de Faria MJ, Moreira EG, Gerardin DC. Maternal exposure to the antidepressant fluoxetine impairs sexual motivation in adult male mice. Pharmacology, Biochemistry, and Behavior. 2008;**90**:416-419

[91] Harris SS, MacIag D, Simpson KL, Lin RCS, Paul IA. Dose-dependent effects of neonatal SSRI exposure on adult behavior in the rat. Brain Research. 2012;**1429**:52-60

[92] Maciag D, Simpson KL, Coppinger D, Lu Y, Wang Y, Lin RC, et al. Neonatal antidepressant exposure has lasting effects on behavior and serotonin circuitry. Neuropharmacology. 2006;**31**:47-57

[93] Rayen I, Steinbusch HW, Charlier TD, Pawluski JL. Developmental fluoxetine exposure and prenatal stress alter sexual differentiation of the brain and reproductive behavior in male offspring. Psychoneuroendocrinology. 2013;**38**:1618-1629

[94] Chan JSW, Snoeren EMS, Cuppen E, Waldinger MD, Olivier B, Oosting RS. The serotonin transporter plays an important role in male sexual behavior: A study in serotonin transporter knockout rats. The Journal of Sexual Medicine. 2011;**8**(1):97-108

[95] Cagiano R, Flace P, Bera I, Maries L, Cioca G, Sabatini R, et al. Neurofunctional effects in rats prenatally exposed to fluoxetine. European Review for Medical and Pharmacological Sciences. 2008;**12**(3):137-148

[96] Rayen I, Steinbusch HW, Charlier TD, Pawluski JL. Developmental fluoxetine exposure facilitates sexual behavior in female offspring. Psychopharmacologia. 2014;**231**:123-133

[97] Grahame-Smith DG. Serotonin function in affective disorders. Acta Psychiatrica Scandinavica. Supplementum. 1989;**350**:7-12

[98] Ansorge MS, Zhou M, Lira A, Hen R, Gingrich JA. Early-life blockade of the 5-HT transporter alters emotional behavior in adult mice. Science. 2004;**306**(5697):879-881

[99] Rebello TJ, Yu Q, Goodfellow NM, Caffrey Cagliostro MK, Teissier A, Morelli E, et al. Postnatal day 2 to 11 constitutes a 5-HT-sensitive period impacting adult mPFC function. The Journal of Neuroscience. 2014;**34**(37):12379-12393. DOI: 10.1523/JNEUROSCI.1020-13.2014

[100] Sarkar A, Chachra P, Vaidya VA. Postnatal fluoxetine-evoked anxiety is prevented by concomitant 5-HT2A/Creceptor blockade and mimicked by postnatal 5-HT2A/Creceptor stimulation. Biological Psychiatry. 2014;**76**(11):858-868

[101] Maciag D, Williams L, Coppinger D, Paul IA. Neonatal citalopram exposure produces lasting changes in behavior which are reversed by adult imipramine treatment. European Journal of Pharmacology. 2006;**532**(3):265-269

[102] Lee LJ, Lee LJH. Neonatal fluoxetine exposure alters motor performances of adolescent rats. Developmental Neurobiology. 2012;**72**(8):1122-1132

[103] Karpova NN, Lindholm J, Pruunsild P, Timmusk T, Castrén E. Long-lasting behavioural and molecular alterations induced by early postnatal fluoxetine exposure

are restored by chronic fluoxetine treatment in adult mice. European Neuropsychopharmacology. 2009;**19**(2):97-108

[104] Bairy KL, Madhyastha S, Ashok KP, Bairy I, Malini S. Developmental and behavioral consequences of prenatal fluoxetine. Pharmacology. 2007;**79**:1-11

[105] Zohar I, Shoham S, Weinstock M. Perinatal citalopram does not prevent the effect of prenatal stress on anxiety, depressive-like behaviour and serotonergic transmission in adult rat offspring. The European Journal of Neuroscience. 2015;**43**(4):590-600

[106] Hansen H, Sanchez C, Meier E. Neonatal administration of the selective serotonin reuptake inhibitor Lu 10-134-C increases forced swimming-induced immobility in adult rats: A putative animal model of depression? The Journal of Pharmacology and Experimental Therapeutics. 1997;**283**(3):1333-1341

[107] Toffoli LV, Rodrigues GM, Oliveira JF, Silva AS, Moreira EG, Pelosi GG, et al. Maternal exposure to fluoxetine during gestation and lactation affects the DNA methylation programming of rat's offspring: Modulation by folic acid supplementation. Behavioural Brain Research. 2014;**265**:142-147

[108] Knaepen L, Rayen I, Charlier TD, Fillet M, Houbart V, van Kleef M, et al. Developmental fluoxetine exposure normalizes the long-term effects of maternal stress on post-operative pain in Sprague-Dawley rat offspring. PLoS One. 2013;**8**(2):e57608

[109] Glover ME, Pugh PC, Jackson NL, Cohen JL, Fant AD, Akil H, et al. Early-life exposure to the SSRI paroxetine exacerbates depression-like behavior in anxiety/depression-prone rats. Neuroscience. 2015;**284**:775-797

[110] Boulle F, Pawluski JL, Homberg JR, Machiels B, Kroeze Y, Kumar N, et al. Developmental fluoxetine exposure increases behavioral despair and alters epigenetic regulation of the hippocampal BDNF gene in adult female offspring. Hormones and Behavior. 2016;**80**:47-57

[111] Coleman FH, Christensen HD, Gonzalez CL, Rayburn WF. Behavioral changes in developing mice after prenatal exposure to paroxetine (Paxil). American Journal of Obstetrics and Gynecology. 1999;**181**:1166-1171

[112] McAllister BB, Kiryanova V, Dyck RH. Behavioural outcomes of perinatal maternal fluoxetine treatment. Neuroscience. 2012;**226**:356-366

[113] Krishnan V, Nestler E. Animal models of depression: Molecular perspectives Vaishnav. Current Topics in Behavioral Neurosciences. 2011;**7**:121-147

[114] Porsolt RD, Le Pichon M, Jalfre M. Depression: A new animal model sensitive to antidepressant treatments. Nature. 1977;**266**(5604):730-732

[115] Glover ME, Clinton SM. Of rodents and humans: A comparative review of the neurobehavioral effects of early life SSRI exposure in preclinical and clinical research. International Journal of Developmental Neuroscience. 2016;**51**:50-72

[116] Hilakivi L, Hilakivi I. Increased adult behavioral "despair" in rats neonatally exposed to desipramine or zimeldine: An animal model of depression? Pharmacology, Biochemistry, and Behavior. 1987;**28**(3):367-369

[117] Velazquez-Moctezuma J, Diaz RO. Neonatal treatment with clomipramine increased immobility in the forced swim test: An attribute of animal models of depression. Pharmacology, Biochemistry, and Behavior. 1992;**42**(4):737-739

[118] Bhagya V, Srikumar BN, Raju TR, Shankaranarayana Rao BS. The selective noradrenergic reuptake inhibitor reboxetine restores spatial learning deficits, biochemical changes, and hippocampal synaptic plasticity in an animal model of depression. Journal of Neuroscience Research. 2015;**93**(1):104-120

[119] Yang LM, Hu B, Xia YH, Zhang BL, Zhao H. Lateral habenula lesions improve the behavioral response in depressed rats via increasing the serotonin level in dorsal raphe nucleus. Behavioural Brain Research. 2008;**188**(1):84-90

[120] Vazquez-Palacios G, Bonilla-Jaime H, Velazquez-Moctezuma J. Antidepressant effects of nicotine and fluoxetine in an animal model of depression induced by neonatal treatment with clomipramine. Progress in Neuro-Psychopharmacology & Biological Psychiatry. 2005;**29**:39-46

[121] Limón-Morales O, Soria-Fregozo C, Arteaga-Silva M, Vázquez-Palacios G, Bonilla-Jaime H. Altered expression of 5-HT1A receptors in adult rats induced by neonatal treatment with clomipramine. Physiology & Behavior. 2014;**124**:37-44

[122] Mendes-da-Silva C, De Souza SL, Barreto-Medeiros JM, De Freitas-Silva SR, Costa Antunes DE, Urbano Cunha AD, et al. Neonatal treatment with fluoxetine reduces depressive behavior induced by forced swim in adult rats. Arquivos de Neuro-Psiquiatria. 2002;**60**(4):928-931

[123] Liu M-Y, Yin C-Y, Zhu L-J, Zhu X-H, Xu C, Luo C-X, et al. Sucrose preference test for measurement of stress-induced anhedonia in mice. Nature Protocols. 2018;**13**(7):1686-1698

[124] Popa D, Lena C, Alexandre C, Adrien J. Lasting syndrome of depression produced by reduction in serotonin uptake during postnatal development: Evidence from sleep, stress, and behavior. The Journal of Neuroscience. 2008;**28**(14):3546-3554

[125] Francis-Oliveira J, Ponte B, Barbosa APM, Veríssimo LF, Gomes MV, Pelosi GG, et al. Fluoxetine exposure during pregnancy and lactation: Effects on acute stress response and behavior in the novelty-suppressed feeding are age and gender-dependent in rats. Behavioural Brain Research. 2013;**252**:195-203

[126] van Bodegom M, Homberg JR, Henckens MJAG. Modulation of the hypothalamic-pituitary-adrenal axis by early life stress exposure. Frontiers in Cellular Neuroscience. 2017;**11**:1-33

[127] Daniels WMU, Pietersen CY, Carstens ME, Stein DJ. Maternal separation in rats leads to anxiety-like behavior and a blunted ACTH response and altered neurotransmitter levels in response to a subsequent stressor. Metabolic Brain Disease. 2004;**19**:3-14

[128] Houwing DJ, Ramsteijn AS, Riemersma IW, Olivier JDA. Maternal separation induces anhedonia in female heterozygous serotonin transporter knockout rats. Behavioural Brain Research. 2019;**356**:204-207

[129] Lee JH, Kim HJ, Kim JG, Ryu V, Kim BT, Kang DW, et al. Depressive behaviors and decreased expression of serotonin reuptake transporter in rats that experienced neonatal maternal separation. Neuroscience Research. 2007;**58**(1):32-39

[130] Wei L, David A, Duman RS, Anisman H, Kaffman A. Early life stress increases anxiety-like behavior in Balbc mice despite a compensatory increase in levels of postnatal maternal care. Hormones and Behavior. 2010;**57**:396-404

[131] Schmauss C, Lee-McDermott Z, Medina LR. Trans-generational effects

of early life stress: The role of maternal behavior. Scientific Reports. 2014;**4**:1-11

[132] Gemmel M, Kokras N, Dalla C, Pawluski JL. Perinatal fluoxetine prevents the effect of pre-gestational maternal stress on 5-HT in the PFC, but maternal stress has enduring effects on mPFC synaptic structure in offspring. Neuropharmacology. 2018;**128**:168-180

[133] Rayen I, Steinbusch HWM, Charlier TD, Pawluski JL. Developmental fluoxetine exposure and prenatal stress alter sexual differentiation of the brain and reproductive behavior in male rat offspring. Psychoneuroendocrinology. 2013;**38**(9):1618-1629

[134] Boulle F, Pawluski JL, Homberg JR, Machiels B, Kroeze Y, Kumar N, et al. Prenatal stress and early-life exposure to fluoxetine have enduring effects on anxiety and hippocampal BDNF gene expression in adult male offspring. Developmental Psychobiology. 2016;**58**(4):427-438

[135] Salari AA, Fatehi-Gharehlar L, Motayagheni N, Homberg JR. Fluoxetine normalizes the effects of prenatal maternal stress on depression- and anxiety-like behaviors in mouse dams and male offspring. Behavioural Brain Research. 2016;**311**:354-367

Chapter 5

Orexin 2 Receptor Antagonists from Prefrontal Cortical Circuitry to Rodent Behavioral Screens

Gerard J. Marek, Stephen Chaney and Mark J. Benvenga

Abstract

Orexin is a neuropeptide contained in neurons from several hypothalamic nuclei that project throughout the forebrain analogously to monoamines synthesized by brainstem nuclei. Orexin, like 5-hydroxytryptamine (5-HT), norepinephrine (NE), dopamine (DA), histamine and acetylcholine (ACh) exerts prominent effects on the sleep-wake cycle of all mammals. Activation of the orexin$_2$ receptor appears to induce spontaneous excitatory synaptic currents (EPSCs) on layer V pyramidal neurons due to release of glutamate from thalamocortical terminals similar to activation of 5-HT$_{2A}$ and α_1-adrenergic receptors. Layer V pyramidal cells are the major descending output cell in the prefrontal cortex with projections to the thalamus, striatum, amygdala, brainstem and spinal cord. In keeping with salient modulation of prefrontal cortical physiology, orexin$_2$ receptor antagonists exert similar effects to 5-HT$_{2A}$ receptor antagonists in suppressing hallucinogen (e.g., DOI)-induced head twitches and producing antidepressant-like effects on the differential-reinforcement-of-low-rate 72-s (DRL 72-s) schedule of reinforcement. Currently, there is both negative and some preliminary positive evidence that blocking orexin$_2$ receptors may result in antidepressant efficacy in patients with major depressive disorder. Overall, the treatment of mood disorders is an additional potential indication for orexin receptor antagonists beyond simply improving sleep.

Keywords: antidepressant drug screens, excitatory postsynaptic potential currents (EPSCs), DOI-induced head twitches, differential-reinforcement-of-low-rate 72-s (DRL 72-s) behavior, LSN2424100, layer V pyramidal neurons, prefrontal cortex, thalamocortical axons

1. Introduction

Only approximately 50–60% of patients experience an antidepressant response when treated with selective reuptake inhibitors (SSRIs) or serotonin-norepinephrine reuptake inhibitors (SNRIs) [1–3]. Even those patients that do respond often continue to experience residual symptoms such as insomnia and cognitive dysfunction [4–7]. Thus, novel antidepressant medications are needed that treat a broader expanse of symptoms or are effective in patients that have failed several different classes of antidepressants drugs.

The primary well-documented augmentation treatment for depressed patients already on SSRIs or SNRIs are atypical antipsychotics (aripiprazole, quetiapine, risperidone or olanzapine) and less so for mirtazapine/mianserin [8–12]. The common pharmacological action shared by these medications is blockade of 5-HT_{2A} receptors [13]. Blockade of 5-HT_{2A} receptors may also be a key pharmacological feature for most tricyclic antidepressant drugs which explain their greater antidepressant efficacy compared to SSRIs [14–17]. However, side effects especially problematic for augmentation of SSRIs/SNRIs with atypical antipsychotic drugs are weight gain and extrapyramidal symptoms. Thus, discovery of a drug targeted on key neurocircuitry modulated by 5-HT_{2A} receptors is one strategy to develop a novel antidepressant medication.

Given that pathophysiology of mood disorders appears to involve the prefrontal cortex and associated macrocircuits, an obvious candidate brain region to provide a context for 5-HT_{2A} receptor blockade at augmenting the effects of SSRIs/SNRIs is the prefrontal cortex [18–21]. In particular, layer V pyramidal neurons can effectively modulate important cortical circuits (including corticothalamic, corticostriatal, cortico-amydalar and cortico-brainstem) that impact mood, cognition/executive function, sleep and appetite [22, 23]. One aspect of 5-HT_{2A} receptor function largely restricted to layer V pyramidal cells is increasing the frequency of spontaneous excitatory postsynaptic currents/potentials (EPSC/EPSPs) onto the dendritic branches [24]. This effect appears to be mediated by AMPA receptor stimulation of directly on the layer V pyramidal cells [24, 25]. Lesion studies have suggested that 5-HT_{2A} receptor activation is releasing glutamate from thalamocortical terminals arising from the "non-specific" midline and intralaminar thalamic nuclei [26, 27]. There appear to be hot spots in layer I and layer Va where focal 5-HT-induced release of glutamate sensitive to the sodium channel blocker tetrodotoxin (TTX) occurs, although an amplification of postsynaptic currents, including TTX-sensitive sodium currents [24]. A number of G_i/G_o-coupled GPCRs (including $mGlu_2$, $mGlu_4$, μ-opioid, adenosine A_1 receptors) also suppresses 5-HT- or DOI-induced glutamate release from these terminals [28–33]. Several other G_q/G_{11}-coupled GPCRs (α_1-adrenergic receptors and $mGlu_5$ receptors) also appear to induce glutamate release onto layer V pyramidal neurons that are suppressed by the sodium channel blocker TTX, μ-opioid agonists, and AMPA receptor antagonists [34, 35]. This rich pharmacological modulation of 5-HT_{2A} receptor-mediated electrophysiological effects on dendritic integration for the principle output neurons in the prefrontal cortex provides heuristic promise for drug discovery efforts with respect to major psychiatric disease, including mood disorders and schizophrenia [36, 37].

The increase in spontaneous EPSC/EPSPs upon layer V pyramidal cells induced by 5-HT_{2A} receptor activation may be associated with other electrophysiological, biochemical and behavioral effects involving the medial prefrontal cortex (mPFC). On an electrophysiological level, electrical stimulation of the white matter below the cortex appears to result in an induction of "late" EPSC/EPSPs during washout after application of 5-HT or when the phenethylamine hallucinogen DOI is bath-applied to the cortical slice [38]. These late EPSCs are also suppressed by a range of neurotransmitter receptors that suppress spontaneous 5-HT-induced EPSCs such as agonists for $mGlu_2$, μ-opioid, and adenosine A_1 receptors [30, 32]. There are also some differences between these two electrophysiological responses as NMDA receptor stimulation appears important for the electrical stimulation/DOI-evoked responses unlike the spontaneous 5-HT-induced EPSC/EPSPs [39].

Secondly, systemic DOI administration also induces a range of immediate-early gene-like signals in the prefrontal cortex/neocortex that are also suppressed by activation of $mGlu_2$ autoreceptors and appear dependent on glutamate release from thalamocortical terminals [40–45]. This effect of prefrontal cortical 5-HT_{2A} receptor activation is relatively sparsely studied compared to the electrophysiological or behavioral sequelae.

Third, either systemic administration or local prefrontal cortical administration of agonists for 5-HT_{2A} receptors induces a robust increase in the frequency of head twitches (a behavior infrequently observed under baseline condition) [46, 47]. Agonists or positive allosteric modulators of $mGlu_2$, $mGlu_4$, μ-opioid, adenosine A_1 receptors also suppress DOI-induced head twitches [28, 31, 48–52]. Naturally, these head twitches induced by direct 5-HT_{2A} receptor agonists are also suppressed by a number of antidepressant drugs that potently block 5-HT_{2A} receptors or down-regulate 5-HT_{2A} receptors such as mirtazapine [53], mianserin [54–57], trazodone [55, 58–60], nefazodone [58, 61] and tricyclic antidepressants [55, 57, 62–68] Some of the tricyclic antidepressants are active only with chronic daily administration. While the antidepressant and monoamine oxidase inhibitor (MAOI) tranylcypromine does not directly bind to 5-HT_{2A} receptors, chronic daily administration of this antidepressant has been found to suppress 5-methoxy-N,N-dimethyltryptamine-induced head twitches under conditions associated with a down-regulation of 5-HT_{2A} receptors [63]. The clinical lore regarding μ-opioid receptor agonists and potential antidepressant action is intriguing in light of effects for this class of drugs on DOI-induced head twitches have been discussed elsewhere [36].

Finally, an argument was advanced recently that the basis for detecting antidepressant-like drug effects on the operant differential-reinforcement-of-low-rate 72-s (DRL 72-s) schedule may be related to the biology of a range of neurotransmitter systems that interact with the 5-HT_{2A} receptor in the prefrontal cortex to modulate motor impulsivity [69, 70]. As expected from the similar effects of 5-HT_{2A} receptor antagonists compared to $mGlu_2$ receptor positive allosteric modulators (PAMs) and also to adenosine A_1 receptor agonists for the prefrontal electrophysiology discussed above, 5-HT_{2A} receptor antagonists, $mGlu_2$ receptor PAMs and adenosine A_1 receptor agonists all test similar to known antidepressant drugs in rats performing under the DRL 72-s schedule [51, 71–77].

The underlying thesis of this chapter is that understanding how other neurotransmitter systems interact with 5-HT_{2A} receptors in the medial prefrontal cortex on an electrophysiological, biochemical and behavioral scale may help discover novel antidepressant drugs. Orexin (OX) receptor agonists/antagonists appear to be one such neurotransmitter system that interacts with critical biological aspects of 5-HT_{2A} receptor activation/blockade in thalamocortical pathways influencing the principle output (layer V pyramidal cells) of the prefrontal cortex in a manner suggesting that OX_2 receptor antagonists are putative antidepressant medications.

2. Orexin-2 receptor blockade and putative antidepressant action

The orexins are two peptide neurotransmitters produced in several nuclei within the lateral hypothalamus which are intimately involved in arousal and reward [78]. The name "orexin" was originally coined from the Greek word "orexis" when the orexin/hypocretin peptides were studied for effects on appetite. However, the more salient biological aspect of the orexin system later was realized to be altering sleep and arousal. More specifically, mutations of genes for the orexin-2 (OX_2) receptor, orexin peptides, and loss of orexin-containing hypothalamic cell bodies were demonstrated to be the genetic cause of narcolepsy in canines, mice and humans. The first approved medication targeting the orexin system, suvorexant, blocks both orexin-1 (OX_1) and OX_2 receptors as a dual orexin receptor antagonist (DORA) and is indicated for the treatment of insomnia [78, 79]. Several other DORAs have been shown to be efficacious in treating primary insomnia [80–82]. The overlapping and diverging distribution for the OX_1 and OX_2 mRNA and protein has inspired several decades of past/ongoing research exploring these receptors for sleep, arousal, feeding, alcohol and drug self-administration, stress, anxiety and depression models [83]. The involvement of OX_2 receptors in arousal together with the presence of OX_2 receptor mRNA in the non-specific midline and intralaminar thalamic nuclei and the interactions of the orexin system with brainstem nuclei with overlapping monoamine projections makes the OX2 receptor an especially interesting target for mood disorder therapeutics [78, 83]. As discussed below, OX_2 or hypocretin-2 receptor blockade appears to be a mechanism of action that provides a means of testing the hypothesis discussed above where a drug appropriately modifying multiple levels of biological effects for 5-HT_{2A} receptor activation in the mPFC would be a putative antidepressant medication.

Electrophysiological effects of OX_2 receptor activation in the prefrontal cortex appear to parallel certain effects of 5-HT_{2A} receptor activation when recording from layer V pyramidal neurons. The orexin-B (hypocretin-2) peptide was found to increase spontaneous EPSC/EPSPs in layer V pyramidal neurons of the prefrontal cortex that were blocked by postsynaptic AMPA receptor antagonists as well as by TTX and u-opioid agonists on the presynaptic side similar to the case for 5-HT_{2A} receptor stimulation [84]. Experiments to delineate the origin of afferents in the PFC from which orexin induced glutamate release from suggested that the cells of origin were in the midline and intralaminar thalamic nuclei [84]. Further, the relative potency for orexin-B compared to orexin-A (hypocretin-1) at inducing spontaneous OX-induced EPSCs/EPSPs in PFC layer V pyramidal cells is similar to that found in the intralaminar and midline thalamic nuclei with OX_2, not OX_1, receptor responses [84–86]. The tetrodotoxin sensitivity of the orexin-induced EPSCs/EPSPs is in keeping with earlier studies suggesting that thalamocortical projections from these "non-specific" thalamic nuclei associated with arousal were prone to the generation of terminal spikes as previously suggested [87, 88]. This dependence on thalamocortical pathways originating in the midline and intralaminar thalamic nuclei and terminating in layers I and Va of the prefrontal cortex is consistent with features for the spontaneous 5-HT-induced EPSCs/EPSPs [26, 27]. One difference between OX-induced spontaneous EPSCs and 5-HT-induced EPSCS is that OX does not appear to induce postsynaptic depolarization (consistent with absence of OX_2 mRNA in layer V pyramidal cells) unlike the case for 5-HT_{2A} receptor activation in the majority of layer V pyramidal cells [84, 89]. However, studies characterizing the ability of orexin-B induced EPSCs/EPSPs to be blocked with selective OX_2 receptor antagonists or selective OX_1 receptor antagonists would be useful to unambiguously identify the OX receptor subtype involved in this response.

Limited work has been done exploring effects of OX_2 receptor antagonists on immediate early gene (IEG-like) responses in the prefrontal cortex. However, the OX_2 receptor antagonist LSN2424100 did suppress restraint stress-induced increases in c-Fos protein expression without having any effects on baseline Fos protein expression in the home cage [90]. These effects of the OX_2 receptor antagonist LSN2424100 on restraint stress-induced increases Fos expression in the prelimbic cortex are similar to an effect of the $mGlu_2$ receptor agonist LY354740 on restraint stress-induced increases in Fos expression [45]. As discussed above, 5-HT_{2A} receptor agonists induce a number of immediate IEG-like responses in the prefrontal cortex. Activation of $mGlu_2$ receptors appears to suppress the DOI-induced increases in a number of IEG-like responses in the prefrontal cortex [40, 41, 44, 91].

Modulation of 5-HT_{2A} receptor agonist-induced head twitches is a behavioral measure that is suppressed by a range of antidepressants blocking/regulating 5-HT_{2A} receptors as discussed above; these DOI-induced head twitches are also suppressed by the selective OX_2 receptor antagonist LSN2424100 (**Figure 1**). LSN2424100 possesses approximately 200-fold functional OX_2 receptor antagonist activity at both human recombinant OX_2 vs. OX_1 receptors or rat OX_2 vs. OX_1

receptors [90]. Administration of LSN2424100 (10 mg/kg, i.p.) 30 min prior to administration of DOI (3 mg/kg, i.p.) with behavioral observations beginning 5 min later for a 30 min period resulted in over a 67% statistically significant reduction in the frequency of DOI-induced head twitches in CD-1 mice (n = 8/group; **Figure 1**) using conditions/methods/statistical analyses reported elsewhere in greater detail [52]. Head twitches were observed in 8/8 vehicle/DOI treated mice but in only 3/8 LSN2424100/DOI treated mice ($p < 0.05$, Fisher's Exact Test). This experiment demonstrating that a G_q/G_{11}-coupled GCPR OX_2 receptor antagonist (like 5-HT_{2A} receptor antagonists) suppress DOI-induced head twitches fits in with evidence that agonists or positive allosteric modulators of G_i/G_o-coupled GCPRs ($mGlu_2$, $mGlu_4$, adenosine A_1, and μ-opioid receptors) similarly suppress DOI-induce head twitches [28, 31, 48, 50, 52, 92, 93]. Thus, the effects of these drugs on spontaneous EPSCs/EPSPs upon layer V pyramidal neuron apical dendrites in layers I and Va of the prefrontal cortex all produce directionally consistent effects on DOI-induced head twitches [37]. These results imply that adequate orexin, glutamate, adenosine and endogenous opioid release is present from or onto thalamocortical afferents under the in vivo experimental conditions employed to engender salient changes in dendritic integration of the principle output layer V pyramidal cells.

OX_2 receptor antagonists also appear to modulate at least certain aspects of executive function mediated by the prefrontal cortex, namely impulsivity and biasing operant responding for DRL schedules in rodents [69, 90]. The OX_2 receptor antagonist LSN2424100 increased reinforcers obtained and decreased total responses by Sprague-Dawley rats performing under a DRL 72-s schedule of reinforcement (**Figure 2**) [90]. These antidepressant-like responses were largely replicated in wild-type CD-1 mice and OX_1 receptor knockout mice responding on a DRL 36-s schedule of reinforcement rate [90]. However, no changes in the reinforcement rate or response rate

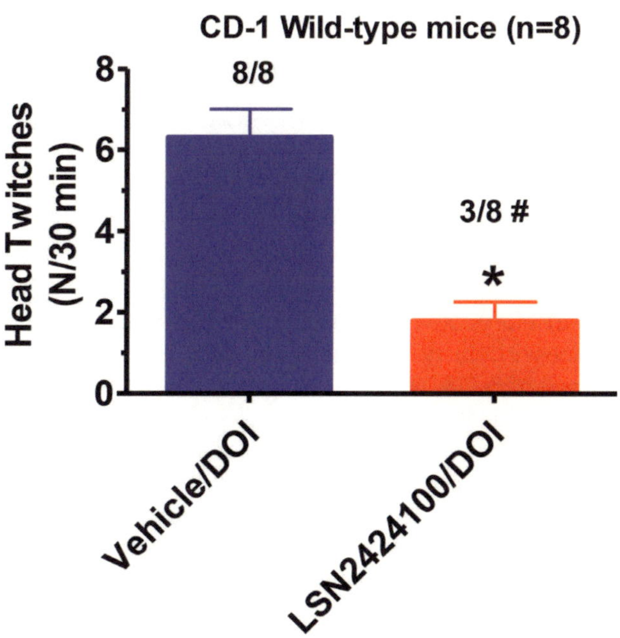

Figure 1.
*The effect of (±)-DOI (3 mg/kg, i.p.) and the selective OX_2 receptor antagonist LSN2424100 (10 mg/kg, i.p.) on head twitches in CD-1 wild-type mice observed for 30 min following drug administration. LSN2424100 was administered 30 min prior to DOI. Each bar represents the mean (± SEM) of eight mice. Significantly different from the mean number of head twitches for the vehicle/DOI group, * $p < 0.05$. Significantly different from the number of mice displaying head twitches for the vehicle/DOI group, # $p < 0.05$ by the Fisher exact test.*

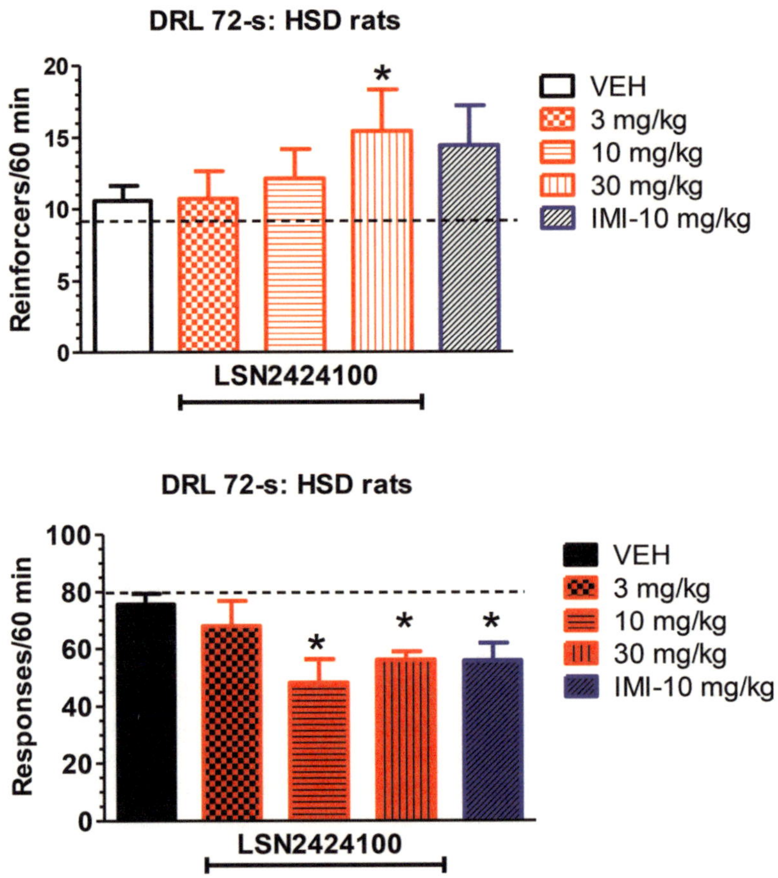

Figure 2.
*The antidepressant-like effect of LSN2424100 on male Sprague-Dawley rats (n = 7) stably performing under a DRL 72-s schedule. The top graph shows the effects of LSN2424100 (3–30 mg, i.p.) and imipramine (10 mg/kg, i.p.) on the number of reinforcers obtained after vehicle/drug was administered 1 hour prior to the daily session. The bottom graph shows the effect of LSN2424100 (3–30 mg, i.p.) and imipramine (10 mg/kg, i.p.) on the total number of responses. The dotted line shows the control reinforcement and response rate and * denotes data points significantly different from control (p < 0.05) (this figure was adapted from data presented by Fitch et al. [90]).*

were observed in OX_2 receptor knockout mice when testing LSN2424100 doses up to twice as large as those used for wild-type and OX_1 receptor knockout mice [90]. A similar antidepressant-like profile was observed in rats, wild-type CD-1 mice, and OX_1 receptor KO mice with the non-selective OX_1/OX_2 receptor antagonist almorexant [90]. In contrast, a selective OX_1 receptor antagonist failed to produce an antidepressant-like response in rats performing on a DRL 72-s schedule or wild type mice or OX_2 receptor knockout mice responding on a DRL 36-s schedule [90]. However, the well-established tricyclic antidepressant drug imipramine tested as expected in these experiments as a positive control (e.g., antidepressant-like effects) in Sprague-Dawley rats, wild-type mice, OX_1 receptor knockout mice, or OX_2 receptor KO mice trained to lever press under a DRL 72-s schedule (rats) or a DRL 36-s (mice) schedule.

3. Clinical trials with orexin receptor antagonists in patients with MDD

Thus far only a single small double-blind, placebo-controlled, diphenhydramine-controlled, parallel group, phase 1b/2a trial of a selective OX_2 receptor antagonist, JNJ-42847922/MIN-202 or seltorexant, has been conducted [94].

Only 47 men and women with a diagnosis of MDD (DSM-IV) were randomized to received either diphenhydramine, 25 mg q.d. (n = 13), seltorexant, 20 mg q.d. (n = 22) or placebo (n = 12) for 10 nights. Sleep polysomnography was also performed to provide objective assessment of improvements on sleep. There were improvements from baseline in the seltorexant treatment group for the HAMD-17 total score (−3.6 points) as well as the HAM-17 adjusted total score accounting for sleep improvement in addition to changes in the HAMD-6 item score (−1.5 points). This resulted in effect sizes of −0.48, −0.55 and − 1.05 for the OX_2 receptor antagonist compared to placebo. However, one caveat is that the subjects assigned to the histamine H_1 receptor antagonist diphenhydramine showed highly comparable improvement compared to placebo as did seltorexant. To answer these questions/concerns, a phase 2b randomized, double-blind parallel group, placebo-controlled, adaptive dose-finding trial for seltorexant adjunctive treatment to antidepressants scheduled to enroll about 280 adult subjects at 85 US, European, Russian and Japanese sites began in September 2017 (NCT03227224).

The only other MDD clinical trial for an OX receptor antagonist was negative [95]. Filorexant (MK-6096), a dual orexin receptor antagonist, was evaluated in a 6-week, double-blind, placebo-controlled, parallel-group phase 2a proof-of-concept trial where subjects with MDD were randomized 1:1 to once-daily oral filorexant 10 mg or matching placebo. Subjects on antidepressants continued to take their prescribed antidepressant for the duration of the trial. This study was stopped after enrolling 129 (40%) of a planned 326 subjects. Less than a 1 point numerical improvement was observed for filorexant compared to placebo using the mean change from baseline to week 6 MADRS total score. Exploratory analyses also failed to reveal statistically significant changes in the Insomnia Severity Index (ISI). Regarding safety, there were no deaths, drug-related serious adverse events (SAEs) and only one discontinuation due to AEs in both treatment groups. There were no other problematic safety issues reported.

This negative filorexant MDD study may be related to an issue of inadequate power as the planned study was designed with 80% power to detect a 3.5-point difference between treatments with a 2-sided 5% level of significance and a fully enrolled trial. However, the enrollment of only 129 subjects while using 61 sites (United States, Canada, Finland, France, Germany, Norway and Sweden) speaks to the recruitment challenges in this study. The dose chosen for this MDD trial appears reasonable based on positive effects reported for filorexant in a phase 2 randomized, double-blind, placebo-controlled adaptive crossover polysomnography dose-ranging study evaluating approximately 80 subjects each at nightly doses of 2.5, 5 and 10 mg [81]. All doses showed significant effects on sleep efficiency and wakefulness after persistent sleep onset while the two higher doses demonstrated significant effects on sleep onset. Filorexant was also well tolerated in this insomnia trial as well [81].

Preclinical results suggest that the combined OX_1/OX_2 receptor antagonism should not have compromised potential antidepressant action in patients with MDD. Namely, the OX_1/OX_2 receptor antagonist almorexant acted similarly to the OX_2 receptor antagonist LSN2424100 and the known tricyclic antidepressant imipramine in rats and mice performing on DRL 72-s or DRL 36-s schedules [90]. In addition, the non-selective OX receptor antagonist almorexant also tested similarly to known antidepressants in mice subjected to unpredictable chronic mild stress (UCMS) and then evaluated with the tail suspension test, the resident-intruder test, and the elevated plus maze [96]. However, opposing antidepressant-like and "pro-depressant"-like effects were observed in OX_1 and OX_2 receptor knockout mice, respectively, studied with the forced swim paradigm [97]. In this same study, the selective OX_1 receptor antagonist SB-334867 also exerted an antidepressant like effect in the forced swim test. No data has been published suggesting that selective OX_2 receptor antagonists test as antidepressants in rodent forced swim tests. Nevertheless, the balance of data are consistent with the hypothesis that adequate blockade of both OX_1 and OX_2 receptors, or OX_2 receptors alone, should improve depressive symptoms in patients with MDD.

4. Conclusions

Activation of 5-HT_{2A} receptors or OX_2 receptors appears to induce glutamate release from thalamocortical terminals with cell bodies originating in the midline and intralaminar thalamic nuclei when recording from prefrontal cortical layer V pyramidal neurons (**Figure 3**). This 5-HT and orexin-B-induced glutamate release appears to dependent action potentials in the presynaptic terminals judging from the TTX-induced blockade of the 5-HT- or orexin-induced EPSC/EPSPs as

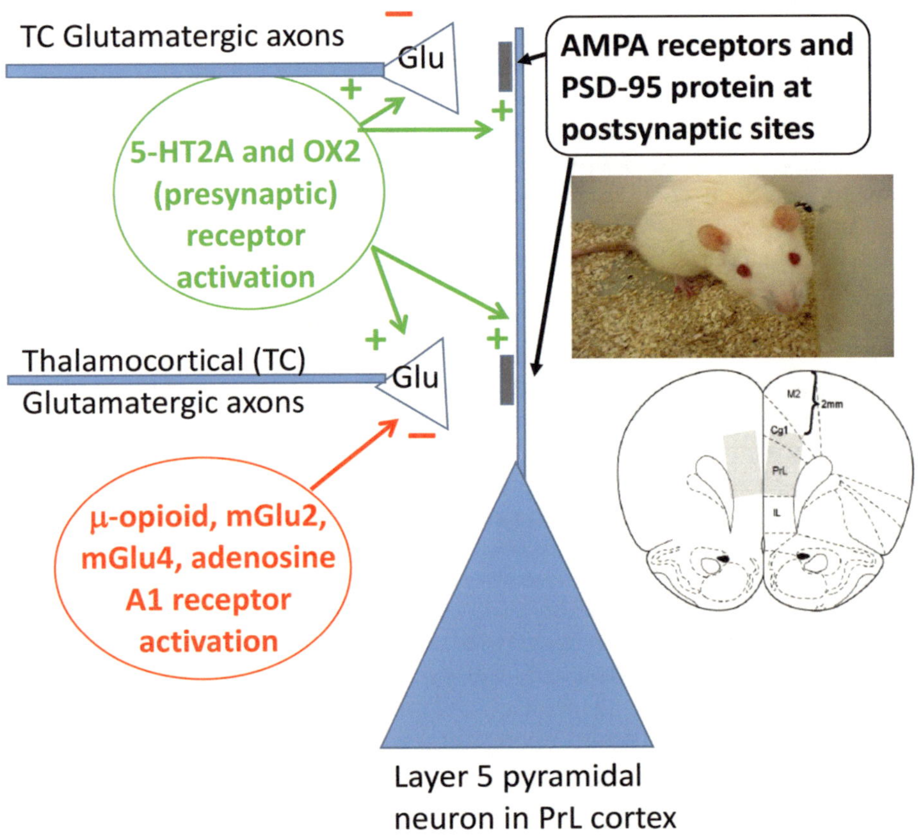

Figure 3.
The model where activation of 5-HT_{2A} or OX_2 receptors depolarizes and releases glutamate from non-specific thalamocortical inputs to layer I and Va of the apical dendrites from layer V pyramidal neurons. The majority of 5-HT_{2A} receptors, apart from a minority of presynaptic receptors and those on GABAergic interneurons, are present on and also directly depolarize layer V pyramidal neurons. Other glutamatergic receptors ($mGlu_2$ and $mGlu_4$), μ-opioid receptors and adenosine A_1 receptors that suppress the EPSCs/EPSPs induced by activation of 5-HT_{2A} and OX_2 receptors appear to be present on non-specific thalamocortical afferents. This circuitry (with additional positive modulator receptor such as $mGlu_5$ and NK_3 receptors and also additional negative modulators such as β_2-adrenergic receptors) appears to underlie a similar valence of action for all these receptors for a behavior mediated by activation of 5-HT_{2A} receptors in the prefrontal cortex, DOI-induced head twitches. This circuitry also appears to underlie impulsive behavior (DRL 72-s behavior) where a similar valence of GPCR mediated effects appears to drive antidepressant-like effects on this screening behavior as DOI-induced head twitches and 5-HT-induced EPSCs.

suggested previously for non-specific thalamocortical axons. Apical dendritic layer V pyramidal AMPA receptors appear to be activated postsynaptic to the thalamic terminals. The 5-HT or DOI-induced spontaneous EPSCs/EPSPs or DOI/electrically evoked EPSC/EPSPs also appear suppressed by $mGlu_2$, $mGlu_4$, adenosine A_1, 5-$HT_{1\text{-like}}$ and β_2-adrenergic receptors.

Future work is required to establish that orexin-B-induced glutamate release from non-specific thalamic afferents is also suppressed by $mGlu_2$, $mGlu_4$, adenosine A_1, 5-$HT_{1\text{-like}}$ and β_2-adrenergic receptors. Blockade of OX_2 and 5-HT_{2A} receptors also both appear to suppress DOI-induced head twitches, a behavioral response that appears to be mediated by activation of prefrontal cortical 5-HT_{2A} receptors. A selective OX_2 receptor antagonist tested similar to the tricyclic antidepressant imipramine in rats and mice responding under an operant DRL 72-s schedule of reinforcement. Another question for future preclinical research with rodent DRL behavior is whether blockade of OX_2 receptors is additive/synergistic with tricyclic antidepressants or SSRIs in the same manner as blockade of 5-HT_{2A} receptors. The ongoing clinical antidepressant trial with the OX_2 receptor antagonist seltorexant are important to understanding whether the circuitry involving orexin-containing cells in the hypothalamus together with orexin-containing axon terminals in the intralaminar and midline thalamic nuclei and the prefrontal cortex are necessary and sufficient by themselves to augment the antidepressant effects of tricyclic antidepressants and SSRIs. If this ongoing and other clinical antidepressant trials with selective OX_2 receptor antagonists or additional adequately powered clinical trials testing OX_1/OX_2 receptor antagonists are negative, then future work will be required to begin to ask whether additional actions of OX_2 receptor antagonists in other circuitry are functionally opposed to the brainstem/thalamic/prefrontal cortical circuits.

Acknowledgements

The present manuscript was not supported by either Astellas or Lundbeck.

Conflict of interest

The authors were previously employed by Eli Lilly.

Author details

Gerard J. Marek[1*], Stephen Chaney[2] and Mark J. Benvenga[3]

1 Astellas Pharma Global Development Inc., Northbrook, IL, USA

2 Eli Lily Research Laboratories, Indianapolis, IN, USA

3 Lundbeck, Sacramento, CA, USA

*Address all correspondence to: gerard.marek@astellas.com

References

[1] Bradley AJ, Lenox-Smith AJ. Does adding noradrenaline reuptake inhibition to selective serotonin reuptake inhibition improve efficacy in patients with depression? A systematic review of meta-analysis and large randomized pragmatic trials. Journal of psychopharmacology (Oxford, England). 2013;**27**:740-758

[2] Cipriani A, Furukawa TA, Salanti G, Geddes JR, Higgins JP, Churchill R, et al. Comparative efficacy and acceptability of 12 new-generation antidepressants: A multiple-treatments meta-analysis. Lancet. 2009;**373**:746-758

[3] Papakostas GI, Charles D, Fava M. Are typical starting doses of the selective serotonin reuptake inhibitors sub-optimal? A meta-analysis of randomized, double-blind, placebo-controlled, dose-finding studies in major depressive disorder. The World Journal of Biological Psychiatry. 2010;**11**:300-307

[4] Mayers AG, Baldwin DS. Antidepressants and their effect on sleep. Human Psychopharmacology. 2005;**20**:533-539

[5] Nakano Y, Baba H, Maeshima H, Kitajima A, Sakai Y, Baba K, et al. Executive dysfunction in medicated, remitted state of major depression. Journal of Affective Disorders. 2008;**111**:46-51

[6] Paelecke-Habermann Y, Pohl J, Leplow B. Attention and executive function in remitted major depression patients. Journal of Affective Disorders. 2005;**89**:125-135

[7] Winokur A, Gary KA, Rodner S, Rae-Red C, Fernando AT, Szuba MP. Depression, sleep physiology, and antidepressant drugs. Depression and Anxiety. 2001;**14**:19-28

[8] Blier P, Gobbi G, Turcotte JE, de Montigny C, Boucher N, Hebert C, et al. Mirtazapine and paroxetine in major depression: A comparison of monotherapy versus their combination from treatment initiation. European Neuropsychopharmacology. 2009;**19**:457-465

[9] Carpenter LL, Yasmin S, Price LH. A double-blind placebo-controlled study of antidepressant augmentation with mirtazapine. Biological Psychiatry. 2002;**51**:183-188

[10] Ferreri M, Lavergne F, Berlin I, Payan C, Peuch AJ. Benefits from mianserin augmentation of fluoxetine in patients with major depression non-responders to fluoxetine alone. Acta Psychiatrica Scandinavica. 2001;**103**:66-72

[11] Han C, Wang S-M, Kato M, Lee S-J, Patkar AA, Masand PS, et al. Second-generation antipsychotics in the treatment of major depressive disorder: Current evidence. Expert Review of Neurotherapeutics. 2013;**13**:851-874

[12] Nelson JC, Papakostas GI. Atypical antipsychotic augmentation in major depressive disorders: A meta-analysis of placebo-controlled randomized trials. The American Journal of Psychiatry. 2009;**166**:980-991

[13] Marek GJ, Carpenter LL, McDougle CJ, Price LH. Synergistic action of 5-HT_{2A} antagonists and selective serotonin reuptake inhibitors in neuropsychiatric disorders. Neuropsychopharmacology. 2003;**28**:402-412

[14] Marek GJ. Regulation of rat cortical 5-$hydroxytryptamine_{2A}$-receptor mediated electrophysiological responses by repeated daily treatment with electroconvulsive shock or imipramine.

European Neuropsychopharmacology. 2008;**18**:498-507

[15] Marek GJ. Cortical 5-hydroxytryptamine$_{2A}$-receptor mediated excitatory synaptic currents in the rat following repeated daily fluoxetine administration. Neuroscience Letters. 2008;**438**:312-316

[16] DUAG. Citalopram: Clinical effect profile in comparison with clomipramine—A controlled multicenter study. Psychopharmacology. 1986;**90**:131-138

[17] DUAG. Paroxetine: A selective serotonin reuptake inhibitor showing better tolerance, but weaker antidepressant effect than clomipramine in a controlled multicenter study. Journal of Affective Disorders. 1990;**18**:289-299

[18] Drevets WC. Functional neuroimaging studies of depression: The anatomy of melancholia. Annual Review of Medicine. 1998;**49**:341-361

[19] Drevets WC, Videen TO, Price JL, Preskorn SH, Carmichael ST, Raichle ME. A functional anatomical study of unipolar depression. Journal of Neuroscience. 1992;**12**:3628-3641

[20] Mayberg HS. Limbic-cortical dysregulation: A proposed model of depression. Journal of Neuropsychiatry & Clinical Neurosciences. 1997;**9**(3):471-481

[21] Rajkowska G, Miguel-Hidalgo JJ, Wei J, Dilley G, Pittman SD, Meltzer HY, et al. Morphometric evidence for neuronal and glia prefrontal cell pathology in major depression. Biological Psychiatry. 1999;**45**:1085-1098

[22] Price JL. Prefrontal cortical networks related to visceral function and mood. Annuals of New York Academy of Sciences. 1999;**877**:383

[23] Price JL, Drevets WC. Neurocircuitry of mood disorders. Neuropsychopharmacology. 2010;**35**:192-216

[24] Aghajanian GK, Marek GJ. Serotonin induces excitatory postsynaptic potentials in apical dendrites of neocortical pyramidal cells. Neuropharmacology. 1997;**36**(3/4):589-599

[25] Zhang C, Marek GJ. AMPA receptors involvement in 5-hydroxytryptamine$_{2A}$ receptor-mediated prefrontal cortical excitatory synaptic currents and DOI-induced head shakes. Progress in Neuro-Psychopharmacology & Biological Psychiatry. 2008;**32**:62-71

[26] Lambe EK, Aghajanian GK. The role of Kv1.2-containing potassium channels in serotonin-induced glutamate release from thalamocortical terminals in rat frontal cortex. The Journal of Neuroscience. 2001;**21**:9955-9963

[27] Marek GJ, Wright RA, Gewirtz JC, Schoepp DD. A major role for thalamocortical afferents in serotonergic hallucinogen receptor function in the rat neocortex. Neuroscience. 2001;**105**:379-392

[28] Benneyworth MA, Xiang Z, Smith RL, Garcia EE, Conn PJ, Sanders-Bush E. A selective positive allosteric modulator of metabotropic glutamate receptor subtype 2 blocks a hallucinogenic drug model of psychosis. Molecular Pharmacology. 2007;**72**:477-484

[29] Marek GJ, Aghajanian GK. 5-HT-induced EPSCs in neocortical layer V pyramidal cells: Suppression by μ-opiate receptor activation. Neuroscience. 1998;**86**:485-497

[30] Marek GJ, Wright RA, Schoepp DD, Monn JA, Aghajanian GK. Physiological antagonism between 5-hydroxytryptamine$_{2A}$ and group

II metabotropic glutamate receptors in prefrontal cortex. The Journal of Pharmacology and Experimental Therapeutics. 2000;**292**:76-87

[31] Slawinska A, Wieronska JM, Stachowicz K, Marciniak M, Lason-Tyburkiewicz M, Gruca P, et al. The antipsychotic-like effects of positive allosteric modulators of metabotropic glutamate mGlu4 receptors in rodents. British Journal of Pharmacology. 2013;**169**:1824-1839

[32] Stutzman GE, Marek GJ, Aghajanian GK. Adenosine preferentially suppresses serotonin2A receptor-enhanced excitatory postsynaptic currents in layer V neurons of the rat medial prefrontal cortex. Neuroscience. 2001;**105**:55-69

[33] Zhang C, Marek GJ. Group III metabotropic glutamate receptor agonists selectively suppress excitatory synaptic currents in the rat prefrontal cortex induced by 5-hydroxytryptamine$_{2A}$ receptor stimulation. The Journal of Pharmacology and Experimental Therapeutics. 2007;**320**:437-447

[34] Marek GJ, Zhang C. Activation of metabotropic glutamate 5 (mGlu5) receptors induces spontaneous excitatory synaptic currents in layer V pyramidal cells of the rat prefrontal cortex. Neuroscience Letters. 2008;**442**:239-243

[35] Marek GJ, Aghajanian GK. 5-HT$_{2A}$ or α_1-adrenoceptor activation induces excitatory postsynaptic currents in layer V pyramidal cells of the medial prefrontal cortex. European Journal of Pharmacology. 1999;**367**:197-206

[36] Marek GJ, Aghajanian GK. The electrophysiology of prefrontal 5-HT systems: Therapeutic implications for mood and psychosis. Biological Psychiatry. 1998;**44**:1118-1127

[37] Marek GJ. Interactions of Hallucinogens with the Glutamatergic System: Permissive Network Effects Mediated through Cortical Layer V Pyramidal Neurons. Current Topics in Behavioral Neuroscience. Berlin, Heidelberg: Springer; 2017

[38] Aghajanian GK, Marek GJ. Serotonin, via 5-HT$_{2A}$ receptors, increases EPSCs in layer V pyramidal cells of prefrontal cortex by an asynchronous mode of glutamate release. Brain Research. 1999;**825**:161-171

[39] Lambe EK, Aghajanian GK. Hallucinogen-induced UP states in the brain slice rat prefrontal cortex: Role of glutamate spillover and NR2B-NMDA receptors. Neuropsychopharmacology. 2006;**31**:1682-1689

[40] Gewirtz JC, Chen AC, Terwilliger R, Duman RC, Marek GJ. Modulation of DOI-induced increases in cortical BDNF expression by group II mGlu receptors. Pharmacology, Biochemistry, and Behavior. 2002;**73**:317-326

[41] Gonzalez-Maeso J, Ang RL, Yuen T, Chan P, Weisstaub NV, Lopez-Gimenez JF, et al. Identification of a serotonin/glutamate receptor complex implicated in psychosis. Nature. 2008;**452**:93-97

[42] Gonzalez-Maeso J, Weisstaub NV, Zhou M, Chan P, Ivic L, Ang R, et al. Hallucinogens recruit specific cortical 5-HT$_{2A}$ receptor-mediated signalling pathways to affect behavior. Neuron. 2007;**53**:439-452

[43] Scruggs JL, Patel S, Bubser M, Deutch AY. DOI-induced activation of the cortex: Dependence upon 5-HT$_{2A}$ heteroceptors on thalamocortical glutamatergic neurons. The Journal of Neuroscience. 2000;**20**:8846-8852

[44] Wischhof L, Koch M. Pretreatment with the mGlu2/3 receptor agonist LY379268 attenuates DOI-induced impulsive responding and

regional c-Fos protein expression. Psychopharmacology. 2012;**219**:387-400

[45] Menezes MM, Marek GJ, Benvenga MJ, Chaney S, Svensson KA. The mGlu2/3 receptor agonist LY354740 attenuates the restraint-stress induced Fos expression and DOI-induced Fos expression in prefrontal cortex. In: Neuroscience Meeting Planner Society for Neurocience. Chicago, IL: Society for Neuroscience; 2009. pp. 417-423

[46] Canal CE, Morgan D. Head-twitch response in rodents induced by the hallucinogen 2,5-dimethoxy-4-iodoamphetamine: A comprehensive history, a re-evaluation of mechanisms, and its utility as a model. Drug Test Analysis. 2012;**4**:556-576

[47] Willins DL, Meltzer HY. Direct injection of 5-HT2A receptor agonists into the medial prefrontal cortex produces a head-twitch response in rats. The Journal of Pharmacology and Experimental Therapeutics. 1997;**282**:699-706

[48] Gewirtz JC, Marek GJ. Behavioral evidence for interactions between a hallucinogenic drug and group II metabotropic glutamate receptors. Neuropsychopharmacology. 2000;**23**:569-576

[49] Klodzinska A, Bijak M, Tokarski K, Pilc A. Group II mGlu receptor agonists inhibit behavioral and electrophysiological effects of DOI in mice. Pharmacology Biochemistry & Behavior. 2002;**73**:327-332

[50] Marek GJ. Behavioral evidence for μ-opioid and $5\text{-}HT_{2A}$ receptor interactions. European Journal of Pharmacology. 2003;**474**:77-83

[51] Marek GJ. Activation of $adenosine_1$ receptors induces antidepressant-like, anti-impulsive effects on differential reinforcement of low-rate 72-s behavior in rats. The Journal of Pharmacology and Experimental Therapeutics. 2012;**341**:564-570

[52] Benvenga MJ, Chaney S, Baez M, Britton TC, Hornback WJ, Monn JA, et al. Metabotropic glutamate2 receptors play a key role in modulating head twitches induced by a serotonergic hallucinogen in mice. Frontiers in Pharmacology. 2018;**9**:208

[53] Rojoz Z. Effect of co-treatment with mirtazapine and risperidone in animal models of the positive symptoms of schizophrrenia in mice. Pharmacological Reports. 2012;**64**:1567-1572

[54] Blackshear MA, Sanders-Bush E. Serotonin receptor sensitivity after acute and chronic treatment with mianserin. The Journal of Pharmacology and Experimental Therapeutics. 1982;**221**:303-308

[55] Friedman E, Cooper TB, Dallob A. Effects of chronic antidepressant treatment on serotonin receptor activity in mice. European Journal of Pharmacology. 1983;**89**:69-76

[56] Maj J, Rogoz Z, Skuza G, Sowinska H. The effect of repeated administration of imipramine, citalopram and mianserin on responsiveness of central serotonergic, alpha 2-adrenergic and cholinergic system in mice. Polish Journal of Pharmacology and Pharmacy. 1989;**41**:313-319

[57] Ogren SO, Fuxe K, Agnati LF, Gustafsson JA, Jonsson G, Holm AC. Reevalulation of the indoleamine hypothesis of depression. Evidence for a reduction of functional activity of central 5-HT systems by antidepressant drugs. Journal of Neural Transmission. 1979;**46**:85-103

[58] Taylor DP, Carter RB, Eison AS, Mullins UL, Smith HL, Torrente JR, et al. Pharmacology and neurochemistry

of nefazodone, a novel antidepressant drug. Journal of Clinical Psychiatry. 1995;**56**(Suppl 6):3-11

[59] Clements-Jewery S, Robson PA, Chidley LJ. Biochemical investigations into the mode of action of trazodone. Neuropharmacology. 1980;**19**:1165-1173

[60] Cioli V, Corradino C, Piccinelli D, Rocchi MG, Valeri P. A comparative pharmacological study of trazodone, etoperidone and 1-(m-chlorophenyl) piperazine. Pharmacological Research Communications. 1984;**16**:85-100

[61] Nacca A, Guiso G, Fracasso C, Cervo L, Caccia S. Brain-to-blood partition and in vivo inhibition of 5-hydroxytryptamine reuptake and quipazine-mediated behaviour of nefazodone and its main active metabolites in rodents. British Journal of Pharmacology. 1998;**1998**:1617-1623

[62] Wettstein JG, Host M, Hitchcock JM. Selectivity of action of typical and atypical anti-psychotic drugs as antagonists of the behavioral effects of 1-[2,5-dimethoxy-4-iodophenyl]-2-aminopropane (DOI). Progress in Neuro-Psychopharmacology & Biological Psychiatry. 1999;**23**:533-544

[63] Goodwin GM, Green AR, Johnson P. 5-HT_2 receptor characteristics in frontal cortex and 5-HT_2 receptor-mediated head-twitch behavior following antidepressant treatment to mice. British Journal of Pharmacology. 1984;**83**:235-242

[64] Godfrey PP, McClue SJ, Young MM, Heal DJ. 5-hydroxytryptamine-stimulated inositol phospholipid hydrolysis in the mouse cortex has pharmacological characteristics compatible with mediation via 5-HT2 receptors but this response does not reflect altered 5-HT2 function after 5,7-dihydroxytryptamine lesioning or repeated antidepressant treatments. Journal of Neurochemistry. 1988;**50**:730-738

[65] Pawlowski L, Ruczynska J, Gorka Z. Citalopram: A new potent inhibitor of serotonin (5-HT) uptake with central 5-HT-mimetic properties. Psychopharmacology. 1981;**74**:161-165

[66] Pawlowski L, Melzacka M. Inhibition of head twitch response to quipazine in rats by chronic amitriptyline but not fluvoxamine or citalopram. Psychopharmacology. 1986;**88**:279-284

[67] Kawakami Y, Kitamura Y, Araki H, Kitagawa K, Suemaru K, Shibata K, et al. Effects of monoamine reuptake inhibitors on wet-dog shakes mediated by 5-HT2A receptors in ACTH-treated rats. Pharmacology, Biochemistry, and Behavior. 2005;**81**:65-70

[68] Kitamura Y, Araki H, Suemaru K, Gomita Y. Effects of imipramine and lithium on wet-dog shakes mediated by the 5-HT2A receptor in ACTH-treated rats. Pharmacology, Biochemistry, and Behavior. 2002;**72**:397-402

[69] Marek GJ, Day M, Hudzik TJ. The utility of impulsive bias and altered decision making as predictors of drug efficacy and target selection: Rethinking behavioral screening for antidepressant drugs. The Journal of Pharmacology and Experimental Therapeutics. 2016;**356**:534-548

[70] O'Donnell JM, Marek GJ, Seiden LS. Antidepressant effects assessed using behavior maintained under a differential-reinforcement-of-low-rate (DRL) operant schedule. Neuroscience and Biobehavioral Reviews. 2005;**29**:785-798

[71] Marek GJ, Li AA, Seiden LS. Selective 5-hydroxytryptamine2 antagonists have antidepressant-like effects on

differential-reinforcement-of-low-rate 72-second schedule. The Journal of Pharmacology and Experimental Therapeutics. 1989;**250**(1):52-59

[72] Marek GJ, Martin-Ruiz R, Abo A, Artigas F. The selective 5-HT_{2A} receptor antagonist M100907 enhances antidepressant-like behavioral effects of the SSRI fluoxetine. Neuropsychopharmacology. 2005;**30**:2205-2215

[73] Marek GJ, Seiden LS. Effects of selective 5-hydroxytryptamine-2 and nonselective 5-hydroxytryptamine antagonists on the differential-reinforcement-of-low-rate 72-second schedule. The Journal of Pharmacology and Experimental Therapeutics. 1988;**244**(2):650-658

[74] Ardayfio PA, Benvenga MJ, Chaney SF, Love PL, Catlow J, Swanson SP, et al. The 5-hydroxytryptamine2A receptor antagonist R-(+)-a-(2,3-dimethoxyphenyl)-1-[2-(4-fluorophenyl) ethyl-4-piperidinemethanol] (M100907) attenuates impulsivity after both drug-induced disruption (dizocilpine) and enhancement (antidepressant drugs) of differential-reinforcement-of-low-rate 72-s behavior in the rat. The Journal of Pharmacology and Experimental Therapeutics. 2008;**327**:891-897

[75] Fell MJ, Witkin JM, Falcone JF, Katner JS, Perry KW, Hart J, et al. N-(4-((2-(trifluoromethyl)-3-hydroxy-4-(isobutyryl)phenoxy)methyl) benzyl)-1-methyl-1H-imidazole-4-carboxamide (THIIC), a novel metabotropic glutamate 2 potentiator with potential anxiolytic/antidepressant properties: In vivo profiling suggests a link between behavioral and central nervous system neurochemical changes. The Journal of Pharmacology and Experimental Therapeutics. 2011;**336**:165-177

[76] Nikiforuk A, Popik P, Drescher KU, van Gaalen M, Relo A-L, Mezler M, et al. Effects of a positive allosteric modulatory of group II metabotropic glutamate receptors, LY487379, on cognitive flexibility and impulsive-like responding in rats. The Journal of Pharmacology and Experimental Therapeutics. 2010;**335**:665-673

[77] Li AA, Marek GJ, Hand TH, Seiden LS. Antidepressant-like effects of trazodone on a behavioral screen are mediated by trazodone, not the metabolite m-chlorophenylpiperazine. European Journal of Pharmacology. 1990;**177**(3):137-144

[78] Gotter AL, Webber AL, Coleman PJ, Renger JJ, Windrow CJ. International Union of Basic and Clinical Pharmacology. LXXXVI. Orexin receptor function, nomenclature and pharmacology. Pharmacological Reviews. 2012;**64**:389-420

[79] Kuriyama A, Tabata H. Suvorexant for the treatment of primary insomnia: A systematic review and meta-analysis. Sleep Medicine Reviews. 2017;**35**:1-7

[80] Black J, Pillar G, Hedner J, Polo O, Berkani O, Mangialaio S, et al. Efficacy and safety of almorexant in adult chronic insomnia: A randomized placebo-controlled trial with an active reference. Sleep Medicine. 2017;**36**:86-94

[81] Connor KM, Mahoney E, Jackson S, Hutzelmann J, Zhao X, Jia N, et al. A phase II dose-ranging study evaluating the efficacy and safety of the orexin receptor antagonist filorexant (MK-6096) in patients with primary insomnia. The International Journal of Neuropsychopharmacology. 2016;**19**(8):1-10

[82] Murphy P, Moline M, Mayleben D, Rosenberg R, Zammit G, Pinner K, et al. Lemborexant, a dual orexin receptor antagonist (DORA) for the

treatment of insomnia disorder: Results from a Bayesian, adaptive, randomized, double-blind, placebo-controlled study. Journal of Clinical Sleep Medicine. 2017;**13**:1289-1299

[83] Marcus JN, Aschkenasi CJ, Lee CE, Chemelli RM, Saper CB, Yanagisawa M, et al. Differential expression of orexin receptors 1 and 2 in the rat brain. The Journal of Comparative Neurology. 2001;**435**:6-25

[84] Lambe EK, Aghajanian GK. Hypocretin (orexin) induces calcium transients in single spines postsynaptic to identified thalamocortical boutons in prefrontal slice. Neuron. 2003;**40**:139-150

[85] Bayer L, Eggermann E, Saint-Mleux B, Machard D, Jones BE, Muhlethaler M, et al. Selective action of orexin (hypocretin) on nonspecific thalamocortical projection neurons. The Journal of Neuroscience. 2002;**22**:7835-7839

[86] Lambe EK, Liu RJ, Aghajanian GKS. Hypocretin (orexin), and the thalamocortical activating system. Schizophrenia Bulletin. 2007;**33**:1284-1290

[87] Gutnick MJ, Prince DA. Thalamocortical relay neurons: Antidromic invasion of spikes from a cortical epileptogenic focus. Science. 1972;**176**:424-426

[88] Pinault D. Backpropogation of action potentials generated at ectopic axonal loci: Hypothesis that axon terminals integrate local environmental signals. Brain Research Reviews. 1995;**21**:42-92

[89] Araneda R, Andrade R. 5-Hydroxytryptamine$_2$ and 5-Hydroxytryptamine$_{1A}$ receptors mediate opposing responses on membrane excitability in rat association cortex. Neuroscience. 1991;**40**(2):399-412

[90] Fitch TE, Benvenga MJ, Jesudason CD, Zink C, Vandergriff AB, Menezes MM, et al. LSN2424100: A novel, potent orexin-2 receptor antagonist with selectivity over orexin-1 receptors and activity in an animal model predictive of antidepressant-like efficacy. Frontiers in Neuroscience. 2014;**8**(5):1-11

[91] Menezes MM, Santini MA, Benvenga MJ, Marek GJ, Merchant KM, Mikkelsen JD, et al. The mGlu2/3 receptor agonists LY354740 and LY379268 differentially regulate restraint-stress-induced expression of c-fos in rat cerebral cortex. Neuroscience Journal. 2013;**736439**:8

[92] Klodzinska A, Bijak M, Chojnacka-Wojcik E, Kroczka B, Swiader M, Czuczwar SJ, et al. Roles of group II metabotropic glutamate receptor agonists in modulation of seizure activity. Naunyn-Schmiedeberg's Archives of Pharmacology. 2000;**361**:283-288

[93] Marek GJ. Activation of adenosine$_1$ (A_1) receptors suppresses head shakes induced by a serotonergic hallucinogen in rats. Neuropharmacology. 2009;**56**:1082-1087

[94] Recourt K, Van Amerongen G, Jacobs G, Zuiker R, Luthringer R, Van der Ark P, et al. JNJ-42847922/MIN-202, a selective orexin 2 receptor antagonist, demonstrates beneficial effects on mood and sleep with major depressive disorder. European Neuropsychopharmacology. 2017;**27**(Suppl. 4):S866

[95] Connor KM, Ceesay P, Hutzelmann J, Snavely D, Krystal AD, Trivedi MH, et al. Phase II proof-of-concept trial of the orexin receptor antagonist filorexant (MK-6096) in patients with major depressive disorder. The International

Journal of Neuropsychopharmacology. 2017;**20**:613-618

[96] Nollet M, Gaillard P, Tanti A, Girault V, Belzung C, Leman S. Neurogenesis-independent antidepressant-like effects on behavior and stress axis response of a dual orexin receptor antagonist in a rodent model of depression. Neuropsychopharmacology. 2012;**37**:2210-2221

[97] Scott MM, Marcus JN, Pettersen A, Birnbaum SG, Mochizuki T, Scammell TE, et al. Hcrtr1 and 2 signaling differentially regulates depression-like behaviors. Behavioural Brain Research. 2011;**222**:289-294

Chapter 6

The BDNF Loop 4 Dipeptide Mimetic Bis(*N*-monosuccinyl-L-seryl-L-lysine) hexamethylenediamide Is Active in a Depression Model in Mice after Acute Oral Administration

Polina Povarnina, Yulia N. Firsova, Anna V. Tallerova, Armen G. Mezhlumyan, Sergey V. Kruglov, Tatiana A. Antipova, Tatiana A. Gudasheva and Sergey B. Seredenin

Abstract

Low-molecular mimetic BDNF GSB-106, which is a substituted dimeric dipeptide, bis(N-monosuccinyl-L-seryl-L-lysine) hexamethylenediamide, was designed and synthesized in the V. V. Zakusov Research Institute of Pharmacology. The dipeptide activates TrkB, PI3K/AKT, and MAPK/ ERK. GSB-106 is being developed as a potential antidepressant. Its antidepressant activity was detected in a number of rodent tests (0.1–1.0 mg/kg, ip; 0.5–5.0 mg/kg, po). In the present study, GSB-106 was shown to completely eliminate the manifestation of anhedonia in the sucrose preference test and to increase disturbed hippocampal synaptogenesis at acute oral administration (0.1 mg/kg) after 10-day social defeat stress in C57Bl/6 mice.

Keywords: BDNF, depression, dipeptide mimetic GSB-106, anhedonia, synaptogenesis, synaptophysin

1. Introduction

Depression is one of the most widespread mental disorders leading to social disadaptation. According to the WHO data in 2012, there were more than 350 million people suffering from depression. Modern antidepressants require long-term use to achieve a therapeutic effect, while their effectiveness does not exceed 60% [1]. Therefore, the creation of antidepressants with new action mechanisms is regarded as one of the most pressing pharmacology problems.

Fundamental studies established that the pathogenesis of depression was associated with impaired neuroplasticity in the hippocampus and the prefrontal cortex, caused by deficit of brain-derived neurotrophic factor (BDNF) [2]. The clinical

IntechOpen

evidence demonstrates that BDNF levels in blood plasma decrease in depression and resolve as the result of antidepressant therapy [3]. A reduced BDNF content in the prefrontal cortex and hippocampus was found in suicide victims [4]. The antidepressant properties of BDNF were investigated based on its physiological functions. The antidepressant effect of neurotrophin was revealed after central administration in different depression models in rodents [5]. Antidepressant activity was also experimentally established for BDNF mimetic 7,8-dihydroxyflavone, an antagonist of BDNF-specific TrkB receptors [6].

Following the discovery of antidepressant properties of ketamine, over the past decade, a lot of efforts have been made to create new antidepressants with a glutamatergic mechanism of action without ketamine-like side effects. To date, one of them, rapastinel, a modulator of NMDA receptors, is in a third phase of clinical trials [7]. From the theoretical point of view, the most important fact is that antidepressant effect of ketamine and other glutamatergic drugs is mediated by activation of BDNF-TrkB-Akt-mTORC1-signaling cascade which leads to enhanced synaptogenesis [8]. The data proving that mTOR inhibition leads to the disappearance of ketamine antidepressant effects serve as pharmacological confirmation of this conclusion [8].

Thus, both pathophysiological evidence and results of experimental and clinical pharmacological studies demonstrate the feasibility of using the BDNF-TrkB receptor system as a pharmacological target of search for new antidepressants.

A mimetic of the fourth loop of BDNF, GSB-106, which is a substituted dimeric dipeptide, bis(N-monosuccinyl-L-seryl-L-lysine)hexamethylenediamide, was designed and synthesized in the V. V. Zakusov Research Institute of Pharmacology [9]. GSB-106 was established to activate BDNF-specific TrkB receptors and their main post-receptor signaling pathways—PI3K/AKT and MAPK/ERK [10]. GSB-106 demonstrated antidepressant activity at intraperitoneal (i.p.) (0.1–1.0 mg/kg) and oral (0.5–5.0 mg/kg) administration in a number of rodent tests [11, 12]. GSB-106 was also shown to stimulate neurogenesis and synaptogenesis in mouse hippocampus [13, 14].

A tablet dosage form of GSB-106 for oral administration was developed in the Technological Department of the Institute (application for a patent of the Russian Federation 2018107362 from 28 02 2018) to create a drug on the basis of the substance. The dosage form of GSB-106 was shown to be active at doses of 0.01–5.0 mg/kg in forced swimming test in mice and to exceed the "gold standard" of antidepressants, amitriptyline, by intensity of effects [11].

The aim of the current study was to investigate antidepressant effects of the tablet dosage form of GSB-106 at acute administration in a model of depression-like state in mice caused by social defeat stress, in comparison with the widely used antidepressant amitriptyline, having affinity to TrkB receptors according to some data [15]. This model is considered to be one of the most appropriate, since it reproduces the main behavioral and neurobiological signs of depression [16].

2. Materials and methods

2.1 Drugs

GSB-106 (bis(N-monosuccinyl-L-seryl-L-lysine)hexamethylenediamide) was synthesized in the Department of Medicinal Chemistry of the V. V. Zakusov Research Institute of Pharmacology, as described previously [9]. The tablet dosage form of GSB-106 was developed in the Technological Department of the V. V. Zakusov Research Institute of Pharmacology, as described (application for a patent of the

Russian Federation 2018107362 from 28 02 2018). The form contained 1% of GSB-106 and 99% of filler, consisting of lactose, microcrystalline cellulose, polyethylene glycol-polyvinyl alcohol copolymer, and magnesium stearate. The tablet dosage form of amitriptyline was purchased from Federal State Unitary Enterprise "Moscow Endocrine Plant" (Russia).

2.2 Animals

Male adult C57BL/6 mice weighing 18–20 g and male adult outbred mice weighing 25–28 g were used in the study. The animals were obtained from the "Stolbovaya" Central Laboratory for Animal Breeding (Moscow Region, Russia). The animals were housed in a vivarium with a natural change of light regime and free access to standard pelleted food and water. The study was carried out in accordance with the Order of the Ministry of Health Care and Social Development of the Russian Federation No. 199n of 01 04 2016 "Approval Rules of Good Laboratory Practice" and with the Resolution of the Eurasian Economic Commission No. 81 "Concerning adoption of the Good laboratory practice of EAEU in the field of drug circulation." All manipulations with the animals were approved by the Institutional Animal Care and Use Committee of the V. V. Zakusov Research Institute of Pharmacology (Moscow).

2.3 Social defeat procedure

A depressive-like state in C57BL/6 mice was created by chronic stress caused by repeated experiences of social defeats in daily confrontations between males. The social defeat stress was performed as previously reported [6]. The outbred male mice were used as aggressors. The C57BL/6 mice and outbred mice were placed in pairs into experimental cages (28 × 14 × 10 sm), divided in half by a perforated Plexiglas wall, one mouse per compartment. The animals were held in sensory contact in the absence of direct physical interaction for 2 days. Separator was removed for 10 min on day 3 to allow animals opportunity for direct contact. Under these conditions, the larger outbred mouse acted as an "aggressor." The confrontation was stopped before the expiration of 10 min in the case of overly aggressive attacks by the outbred mouse (the bites continued even after the victim mouse had demonstrated a submissive pose). C57BL/6 mice were given daily stress for 10 days as described above, which leads to the development of a depressive-like state, according to the literature [16].

2.4 Design of the experiment

After 10 days of social defeat stress, the social avoidance test was conducted on day 11 to select mice with depressive-like behavior. Then these mice were randomly divided into three groups of eight animals each:

The control (stress) group
The "stress + GSB-106" group
The "stress + amitriptyline" group

2.5 Mice were placed into individual cages

On day 12, mice of the "stress + GSB-106" group were orally administered with GSB-106 in the dosage form at a dose of 0.1 mg/kg (for the active substance), suspended in 1% starch solution; the "stress" group was administered orally with 1% starch solution; the group of "stress + amitriptyline" was administered orally amitriptyline in the tablet form at a dose of 10 mg/kg, suspended in 1% starch solution. Three more groups of mice (eight animals per group) not subjected to stress were formed simultaneously with the beginning of social stress modeling. On day 11, these groups were single orally administered with a 1% starch solution (control group [no stress]), GSB-106 (the group "GSB-106 [without stress]") or amitriptyline (group "amitriptyline [without stress]") in a 1% starch solution, respectively. The dose of GSB-106 was selected based on previously conducted experiments [12]; the one of amitriptyline was based on literature data [17]. The sucrose preference test was performed on day 13. Mice were decapitated; the hippocampus was isolated for subsequent evaluation of the synaptogenesis intensity on day 16. The scheme of the experiment is shown in **Figure 1**.

2.6 The social avoidance test

This test was performed to select mice that developed depressive-like behavior as the result of social defeat stress, as described in [6]. The infrared actimeter from Panlab (Spain) with ActiTrack software (field size 40.0 × 44.0 cm) was used. An individual transparent plastic chamber with holes (8.0 × 8.0 × 8.0 cm) was placed at one end of the field of the actimeter. A mouse was placed into the actimeter for 2.5 min. Then the mouse was returned to the home cage for 30 s. At this time, the "aggressor" unknown for the testing mouse was placed in the plastic chamber, and the testing mouse was placed in the actimeter for 2.5 min again. The duration of the mouse presence in the "interaction zone" (at a distance of 8.0 cm or less from the camera with the aggressor) was estimated. The interaction ratio (IR) was calculated as the ratio of the time spent in the interaction zone in the presence of the aggressor to the time spent in the interaction zone without the aggressor. The value $IR < 1$ was defined as a criterion for depressive-like behavior. Only the mice showing depressive-like behavior in this test (about 90% of the animals) were used in the further experiment.

2.7 The sucrose preference test

Mice were exposed to bottles with water and 1% sucrose solution. The consumption of water and sucrose solution was evaluated by weighing the bottles. The preference of the sucrose solution was calculated by the following formula:

$A_{(s)}/(A_{(s)} + A_{(w)}) \times 100\%$, where $A_{(s)}$ is the amount of consumed sucrose solution, g, and $W_{(w)}$ is the amount of consumed water, g. The reduction of this parameter below the control group level was regarded as the development of stress-induced anhedonia [6]. The test was carried out for 18 h.

2.8 Evaluation of hippocampal synaptogenesis

The content of the presynaptic marker synaptophysin in hippocampus was assessed using Western blot analysis. After defrost, the hippocampal tissue samples were homogenized at 4°C in a glass homogenizer with lysis buffer (50 mM Tris-HCl, 5 mM EDTA, 1 mM dithiothreitol, 1% Triton X-100, pH 7.5) supplemented with a protease inhibitor cocktail (pepstatin, bestatin, leupeptin, and aprotinin, "Sigma-Aldrich," USA), in the ratio of tissue: buffer = 1:10 (weight/volume). Then the samples were incubated at 4°C for 20 min and centrifuged at 15,000 rpm (Allegra® X-12R centrifuge "Beckman Coulter Inc.," USA) at the same temperature for 20 min. The protein levels of the supernatant lysates were determined by the method of Folin-Lowry. The supernatant proteins were separated in a 12% polyacrylamide gel and then transferred onto a polyvinylidene fluoride membrane by

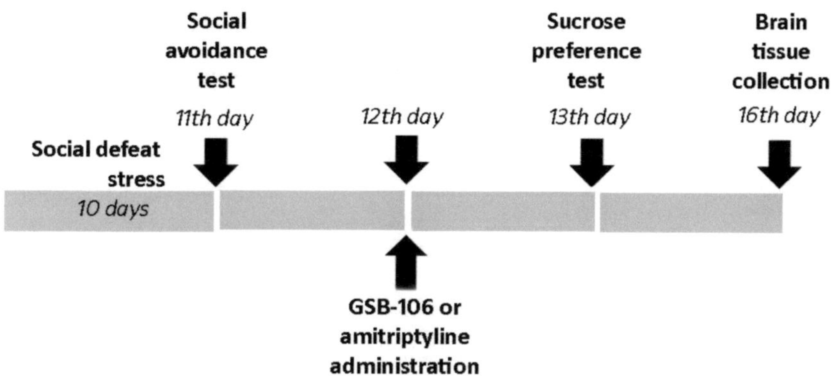

Figure 1.
The scheme of the experiment.

electroelution. The membranes were deactivated with 5% (w/v) nonfat dry milk in Tris buffer containing 1% Tween 20 (TBST) for 1 h. Then, the membranes were treated with primary monoclonal mouse antibodies against synaptophysin ("BD Biosciences," United Kingdom) at a dilution of 1:5000 for 1.5 h, the antibody excess was washed with TBST with 0.5% (w/v) nonfat dry milk, and the membranes were incubated at 37°C with goat antibodies against rabbit IgG ("Santa Cruz Biotechnology," USA, 1:1000), conjugated with horseradish peroxidase, for 1 h. The detection of proteins was performed after washing the secondary antibodies with TBST buffer in the reaction with enhanced chemiluminescence substrates (ECL reagents, Santa Cruz Biotechnology) using the Alliance Q9 gel documenting system (UVITEC, United Kingdom). Densitometry of the obtained images was performed using the GIMP2 program.

2.9 Statistical analysis

The intergroup differences were assessed using one-way analysis of variance ANOVA, followed by post hoc Fisher's LSD test or the Mann-Whitney U test. Differences were considered statistically significant at $p \leq 0.05$; the value of $p < 0.1$ was regarded as a tendency. The data were presented as mean and standard errors of the mean.

3. Results and discussions

One of the main behavioral signs of depression is anhedonia. Anhedonia is a violation of the brain "reward system," it is considered as a key symptom of depression both in the International Classification of Diseases of the tenth revision (ICD-10) and in the Classification of Mental Disorders of the American Psychiatric Association's Diagnostic and Statistical Manual (DSM-5). A common method for assessing anhedonia in animals is the sucrose preference test [6].

In our study the sucrose preference was statistically significantly reduced in the stressed mice (the "control [stress]" group) compared with the intact animals (the "control [without stress]" group) (**Table 1**). GSB-106 statistically and reliably restored the preference of the sucrose solution to the control level. Amitriptyline also restored the preference of the sucrose solution. However, the administration of GSB-106 or amitriptyline to intact animals did not affect the results of this test (**Table 1**).

Groups	n	Amount of consumed 1% sucrose solution, mg	Amount of consumed water, mg	Preference of the 1% sucrose solution, %
Control (without stress)	8	11.4 ± 1.2	2.73 ± 0.5	80.7 ± 3.2
GSB-106 (0.1 mg/kg) (without stress)	8	10.08 ± 0.8	2.14 ± 0.3	82.4 ± 2.8
Amitriptyline (10.0 mg/kg) (without stress)	8	10.02 ± 0.7	3.47 ± 0.1	74.3 ± 6.5
Control (stress)	8	6.67 ± 0.5	2.12 ± 0.2	75.9 ± 2.4*
Stress + GSB-106 (0.1 mg/kg)	8	10.9 ± 1.1	2.4 ± 0.3	81.9 ± 3.1#
Stress + amitriptyline (10.0 mg/kg)	8	13.7 ± 0.9	2.5 ± 0.4	84.8 ± 3.6#

Data are presented as mean ± SEM.
**$p < 0.05$ comparison with the "control (without stress)" group.*
#$p < 0.05$ comparison with the "control (stress)" group (ANOVA followed by the use of the Fisher's LSD method).

Table 1.
The preference of 1% sucrose solution in C57Bl/6 male mice subjected to 10 days of stress, 1 day at acute oral administration of GSB-106 or amitriptyline (test duration—18 h).

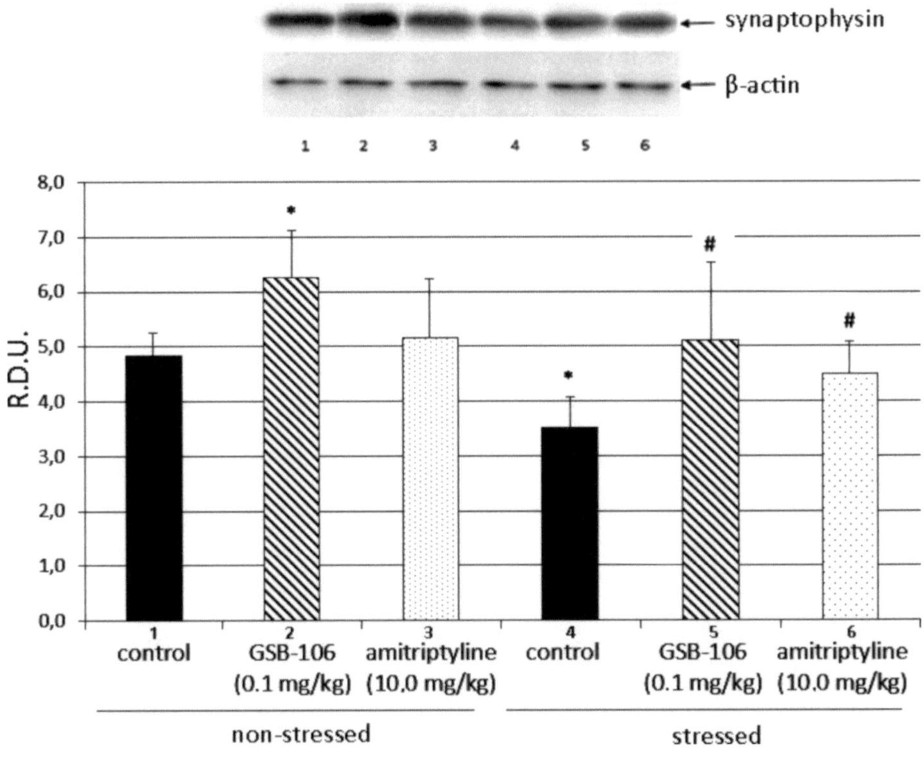

Figure 2.
*The synaptophysin level in the hippocampus of mice on the fourth day after the administration of GSB-106 or amitriptyline. Data are presented as mean ± SEM. Bands: 1, control (without stress); 2, GSB-106 (without stress); 3, amitriptyline (without stress); 4, control (stress); 5, "stress + GSB-106"; 6, "stress + amitriptyline." Note: *$p < 0.05$ compared with the placebo group; #$p = 0.08$ compared with the stress group (Mann-Whitney U test).*

Thus, dipeptide mimetics BDNF GSB-106 completely eliminated the manifestations of anhedonia at acute administration in mice subjected to 10-day social defeat stress.

GSB-106 was previously shown [13] to enhance the synaptophysin content in the hippocampus of mice at chronic administration (21 days). In this study, GSB-106 also caused a statistically significant increase of the synaptophysin content in the hippocampus of the control animals after acute administration (**Figure 2**). In stressed animals, synaptophysin content in the hippocampus was reduced by 30% compared with nonstressed ones. Such a decrease can be considered as a characteristic sign of a depressive-like state, since the hippocampus is the structure most susceptible to pathological changes during depression, as well as the prefrontal cortex, and synaptogenesis impairment is considered as one of the main pathophysiological signs of this disease [2]. The pronounced tendency to restore the level of synaptophysin was observed ($p = 0.08$) at administration of both GSB-106 and amitriptyline to the stressed animals (**Figure 2**).

4. Conclusions

The dipeptide mimetic BDNF GSB-106, like amitriptyline, exhibits anti-anhedonia activity after acute oral administration after 10 days of social defeat stress. The effect of GSB-106 was manifested in doses 100 times smaller than amitriptyline, the drug of comparison.

Conflict of interest

The authors declare no conflict of interest, financial or otherwise.

Funding

This work was supported by the Russian Science Foundation (projects 18-15-00381).

Author details

Polina Povarnina[1], Yulia N. Firsova[2], Anna V. Tallerova[1], Armen G. Mezhlumyan[1], Sergey V. Kruglov[3], Tatiana A. Antipova[3], Tatiana A. Gudasheva[1*] and Sergey B. Seredenin[3]

1 Department of Medicinal Chemistry, V. V. Zakusov Research Institute of Pharmacology, Russia

2 V. V. Zakusov Research Institute of Pharmacology, Moscow, Russia

3 Department of Pharmacogenetics, V. V. Zakusov Research Institute of Pharmacology, Russia

*Address all correspondence to: tata-sosnovka@mail.ru

References

[1] Frodl T. Recent advances in predicting responses to antidepressant treatment. F1000 Research. 2017;**6**:619. DOI: 10.12688/f1000research.10300.1

[2] Wainwright SR, Galea LAM. The neural plasticity theory of depression: Assessing the roles of adult neurogenesis and PSA-NCAM within the hippocampus. Neural Plasticity. 2013;**2013**:805497. DOI: 10.1155/2013/805497

[3] Polyakova M, Stuke K, Schuemberg K, Mueller K, Schoenknecht P, Schroeter ML. BDNF as a biomarker for successful treatment of mood disorders: A systematic & quantitative meta-analysis. Journal of Affective Disorders. 2015;**174**:432-440. DOI: 10.1016/j.jad.2014.11.044

[4] Karege F, Vaudan G, Schwald M, Perroud N, La Harpe R. Neurotrophin levels in postmortem brains of suicide victims and the effects of antemortem diagnosis and psychotropic drugs. Molecular Brain Research. 2005;**136**(1-2):29-37. DOI: 0.1016/j.molbrainres.2004.12.020

[5] Shirayama Y, Chen AC, Nakagawa S, Russell DS, Duman RS. Brain-derived neurotrophic factor produces antidepressant effects in behavioral models of depression. The Journal of Neuroscience. 2002;**22**(8):3251-3261. DOI: 20026292

[6] Zhang JC, Yao W, Dong C, Yang C, Ren Q, Ma M, et al. Comparison of ketamine, 7,8-dihydroxyflavone, and ANA-12 antidepressant effects in the social defeat stress model of depression. Psychopharmacology. 2015;**232**(23):4325-4335. DOI: 10.1007/s00213-015-4062-3

[7] Jelen LA, King S, Stone JM. Alternatives to ketamine in depression: State-of-the-art and future perspectives. Therapeutic Advances Psychopharmacology. 2018;**8**:95-98. DOI: 10.1177/2045125317749456

[8] Abdallah CG, Sanacora G, Duman RS, Krystal JH. Ketamine and rapid-acting antidepressants: A window into a new neurobiology for mood disorder therapeutics. Annual Review of Medicine. 2015;**66**:509-523. DOI: 10.1146/annurev-med-053013-062946

[9] Gudasheva TA, Tarasiuk AV, Pomogaĭbo SV, Logvinov IO, Povarnina P, Antipova TA, et al. Design and synthesis of dipeptide mimetics of the brain-derived neurotrophic factor. Russian Journal of Bioorganic Chemistry. 2012;**38**(3):243-252

[10] Gudasheva TA, Logvinov IO, Antipova TA, Seredenin SB. Brain-derived neurotrophic factor loop 4 dipeptide mimetic GSB-106 activates TrkB, Erk, and Akt and promotes neuronal survival in vitro. Doklady. Biochemistry and Biophysics. 2013;**451**(1):212-214. DOI: 10.1134/S1607672913040121

[11] Povarnina PY, Garibova TL, Gudasheva TA, Seredenin SB. Antidepressant effect of an orally administered dipeptide mimetic of the brain-derived neurotrophic factor. Acta Naturae. 2018;**10**(38):81-84

[12] Seredenin SB, Voronina TA, Gudasheva TA, Garibova TL, Molodavkin GM, Litvinova SA, et al. Antidepressant effect of dimeric dipeptide GSB-106, an original low-molecular-weight mimetic of BDNF. Acta Naturae. 2013;**5**(19):105-109

[13] Gudasheva TA, Povarnina PY, Antipova TA, Seredenin SB. Dipeptide mimetic of the BDNF GSB-106 with antidepressant-like activity stimulates synaptogenesis. Doklady. Biochemistry and Biophysics. 2018;**481**(1):225-227. DOI: 10.1134/S1607672918040130

[14] Gudasheva TA, Povarnina PY, Seredenin SB. Dipeptide mimetic of the brain-derived neurotrophic factor prevents impairments of neurogenesis in stressed mice. Bulletin of Experimental Biology and Medicine. 2017;**162**(4):454-457. DOI: 10.1134/S1607672918040130

[15] Jang SW, Liu X, Chan CB, Weinshenker D, Hall RA, Xiao G, et al. Amitriptyline is a TrkA and TrkB receptor agonist that promotes TrkA/TrkB heterodimerization and has potent neurotrophic activity. Chemistry & Biology. 2009;**16**(6):644-656. DOI: 10.1016/j.chembiol.2009.05.010

[16] Iñiguez SD, Riggs LM, Nieto SJ, Dayrit G, Zamora NN, Shawhan KL, et al. Social defeat stress induces a depression-like phenotype in adolescent male c57BL/6 mice. Stress. 2014;**17**(3):247-255. DOI: 10.3109/10253890.2014.910650

[17] Vilela FC, de Mesquita Padilha M, Alves-Da-Silva G, Soncini R, Giusti-Paiva A. Antidepressant-like activity of *Sonchus oleraceus* in mouse models of immobility tests. Journal of Medicinal Food. 2010;**13**(1):219-222. DOI: 10.1089/jmf.2008.0303